GETTING INTO

Medical School

EIGHTH EDITION

JAMES BURNETT **and** JOE RUSTON

TROTMAN

Getting into Medical School
Eighth edition

This eighth edition published in 2003 in Great Britain
by Trotman and Company Ltd
2 The Green, Richmond, Surrey TW9 1PL
First edition published 1993
Second edition published 1994
Third edition published 1996
Fourth edition published in 1998
Fifth edition published 2000
Sixth edition published 2001
Seventh edition published 2002

British Library Cataloguing in Publication Data
A catalogue record for this book is available from the
British Library.

ISBN 0 85660 873 4

Typeset by Mac Style Ltd, Scarborough, N. Yorkshire

Printed and bound in Great Britain
by Creative Print & Design (Wales) Ltd

CONTENTS

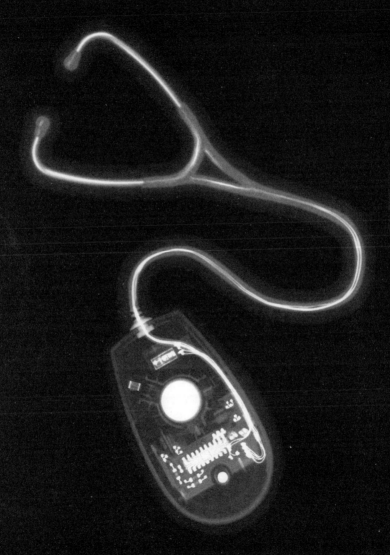

ACKNOWLEDGEMENTS

In order to write this book, I have been able to get help from many sources. Without the help from the medical schools' admissions departments, this book would not exist, and I would like to record my gratitude to all of the people who gave up their time to answer my questions. In particular, I would like to thank Professor Sam Leinster at East Anglia. I am very grateful to Sally Billingham at King Edward's School in Edgbaston, Liz Boddy at Bryanston, Dr Sarah Burnett, ex-Senior Tutor for Admissions at Imperial College, Sheri Newman, Joyce Smart, Andy Long, and Fiona Munro for their help and support.

Finally, I would like to thank the many students and doctors who have provided me with interview questions, factual material and encouragement.

James Burnett

March 2003

For the latest news on medicine and medical schools go to www.mpw.co.uk/getintomed

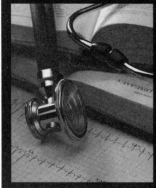
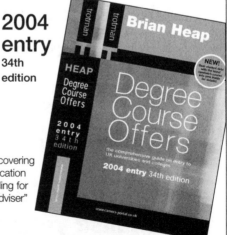

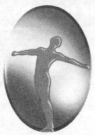

INTRODUCTION TO THE EIGHTH EDITION

Is it easier to get into medical school than it was, say, five years ago? The answer is yes ... and no. On paper, it might seem to be. There are more medical schools – in October 2002 the first students started undergraduate courses at East Anglia and the Peninsula Medical School, and this year students will be able to study at the Hull York Medical School and at the Brighton and Sussex Medical School. In addition to this, there are more undergraduate places at the existing medical schools, and more graduate courses. However, UCAS figures show that the number of people who applied by 15 October 2002 (the deadline for applications for 2003 entry) rose by 28 per cent compared to the previous year, from about 11,000 applicants to over 14,000. Coupled with this, most admissions staff agree that the standard of the candidates is getting better, both in terms of the grades that they achieve and in their awareness of what the selectors are looking for. In other words, the competition for places is tougher. It is worth noting, however, that many of the medical schools – in particular, the new medical schools such as East Anglia – have introduced more flexibility into their admissions processes in order to encourage many more 'non-traditional' entrants.

If getting a place to study medicine was purely a matter of achieving the right grades, the medical schools would demand AAA at A-level and ten A* grades at GCSE, and they would not bother to interview. However, to become a successful doctor requires many skills, academic and otherwise, and it is the job of the admissions staff to try to identify which of the thousands of applicants are the most suitable. It would be misleading to say that anyone, with enough effort, could become a doctor, but it is important for candidates who have the potential to succeed to make the best use of their applications.

Not all of the successful applicants were applying during their final year of A-levels. Some had retaken A-levels, while others had used a gap year to add substance to the UCAS form. Again, it would be wrong to say that anyone who reapplies will automatically get a place, but good candidates should not assume that rejection first time round means the end of their career aspirations.

Gaining a place as a retake student or as a second-time applicant is not as easy as it used to be five years ago, but candidates who can demonstrate genuine commitment alongside the right personal and academic qualities still have a good chance of success if they go about their applications in the right way. The admissions staff at the medical schools tend to be extremely helpful and, except at the busiest times of the year when they simply do not have the time, they will give advice and encouragement to suitable applicants.

Finally, a word about admissions policies. The medical schools make strenuous efforts to maintain fair selection procedures: UCAS forms are generally seen by more than one selector; interview panels are given strict guidelines about what they can (and cannot) ask; and most make available detailed statistics about the backgrounds of the students they interview. Above all, admissions staff will tell you that they are looking for good all-rounders who can communicate effectively with others, are academically able, and are genuinely enthusiastic about medicine: if you think that this sounds like you, then read on!

For the latest news on medicine and medical schools go to www.mpw.co.uk/getintomed

ABOUT THIS BOOK

First of all, a note on terminology. Throughout this guide the term 'medical school' includes the university departments of medicine. Secondly, apologies to readers who have taken Scottish Highers, the International Baccalaureate (or any other qualification) rather than A-levels and AS-levels. Entry requirements have been quoted in A-level terms throughout this book but medical schools are happy to quote requirements in other terms if you ask them. For a general guide to the grades or scores you will need, see the section on the grades you require on page 45.

Would-be doctors face three major obstacles:

■ getting an interview at medical school
■ getting a conditional offer
■ getting the right A-level grades.

The main body of the guide is divided into sections covering each of these three major activities.

Some, but not all, medical schools consider and accept mature candidates (up to the age of about 30), graduates, applicants from abroad, those who studied arts subjects at A-level and those who have had to retake their A-levels. If you are in one of these categories you will need to read pages 56–59.

There are a number of other excellent books on the subject of getting into medical school. Suggestions for further research are included in Appendix D (page 94). The difference between these other books and this one is that this guide is a route map; it tells you the path to follow if you want to be a doctor. To that extent it is rather bossy and dictatorial. We make no apologies for this because we have seen far too many aspiring medical students who took the wrong A-levels, who didn't bother to find work in a hospital and who never asked themselves why they wanted to be a doctor before their interview. Their path into medicine was made unnecessarily difficult because they didn't prepare properly. Finally, the views expressed in this book, though informed by conversation with staff at medical schools and elsewhere, are our own.

James Burnett

March 2003

GETTING AN INTERVIEW

You need an interview because most medical schools issue conditional offers only after the selectors have met you. The evidence that the selector uses when he or she makes the choice to call you for interview or reject you is your UCAS form. Some sections of the form are purely factual (your name, address, exam results, etc). There is also a section where you enter your choice of medical schools. Section 10 gives you an opportunity to write about yourself and there is a space for your headteacher to write a reference describing your strengths and weaknesses. Later in this book, you will find advice on how to fill in these sections and how to influence your referee, but first let's consider what happens, or might happen, to your form.

Typically, a medical school might receive 2500 UCAS forms, almost all of which will arrive in September and October. The forms are copied and distributed to the selectors who have to decide who to recommend for interview. The selectors will usually be busy doctors, and the task of selecting promising candidates means a good deal of extra work for them, on top of the usual demands of their full-time jobs. Most of the candidates will have been predicted grades that will allow them to be considered, but the medical school can only interview, perhaps, 25 per cent of the applicants.

A high proportion of applicants will have good GCSE and AS results and predicted grades at A-level of ABB or higher, and will have undertaken some voluntary work or work-shadowing. In order to decide who should be called for interview, the selectors will have to make a decision based solely on the information provided by you and your school. If you are not called for interview, you will not be offered a place at this medical school. If your UCAS form does not convince the selector that you are the right sort of person to be a doctor, he or she will reject you. However outstanding your personal qualities are, unless the UCAS form is convincing, you will not be called for interview. This part of the guide is designed to maximise your chances of getting the interview even under the worst circumstances.

DECIDING WHERE TO APPLY

There are five medical schools in London, Departments of Medicine at 27 universities outside London, and you can also study medicine at Oxford and Cambridge. The entrance requirements of all medical schools are summarised in Table 1 (page 81).

Oxbridge is in a separate category because, if getting into most medical schools is difficult, entry into Oxford and Cambridge is even more so (the extra hurdles facing students wishing to apply to Oxford or Cambridge are discussed in *Getting into Oxford and Cambridge*, another guide in this series). The general advice given here applies also to Oxbridge but the competition is intense and before you include either university on your UCAS form you need to be confident that you can achieve three A grades at A-level and that you will interview well. You should discuss an application to Oxford or Cambridge with your teachers at an early stage.

Although the UCAS form allows you to apply to six institutions, you may only apply to four medical schools: if you enter more than four, your UCAS form will be returned to you. Under the old system, you were 'advised' to limit your choice to five medical schools but were not, in practice, penalised if you chose six. The new rules are much stricter and you should ignore anyone who advises you that there is no harm in choosing five or even six medical schools.

The question is: what should you do with the other slots? The medical schools will assure you that you can apply for other, non-medical, courses without jeopardising your application to medicine, but I would advise you to think carefully before doing so, for the following reasons:

- There's no point in thinking about alternatives if you really want to become a doctor.
- If you are unlucky and receive no conditional offers for medicine, you could feel yourself obliged to accept an offer from your 'insurance' course. This will make it impossible for you to accept a place for medicine through 'Clearing'. Clearing, in case you haven't heard about it, is the process whereby the places of those who were given conditional offers but didn't get the required A-level grades are shared

out among those who didn't get the conditional offers but did get the grades. The system is described on page 47.

You might find it harder to convince your interviewers that you are completely committed to a career in medicine if you appear to be happy to accept a place to study, say, Chemical Engineering or Archaeology.

The one reason to put two other choices on your form is if you are not prepared to wait a year if your application is unsuccessful, and you intend to enter medicine as a graduate (see page 57).

So, you need to select four medical schools. In deciding which ones to eliminate, you may find the following points helpful.

- If you are worried that you will not achieve ABB/AAB grades the first time round, include at least three schools that accept retake candidates (see Table 1, page 81). The reason for this is that if you make a good impression at interview this year you may not need to face a second interview at your next attempt. You will also be able to show loyalty by applying twice to the same school. Many medical schools will only consider second-time applicants if they applied to them originally.
- A few medical schools do not interview. If you think that you will be a much stronger candidate on paper than in person, it may be advantageous to include these schools. The details of each school's interview policy are shown in Table 1.
- You may be attracted to the idea of being at a university rather than at one of the London medical schools which are not located on the campuses of London University colleges. One reason for this may be the idea that you will find it interesting to mix with students from a wide variety of disciplines and that you will enjoy the intellectual and social cross-fertilisation. The trouble with this theory is that medical students work longer hours than most other students and tend to form a clique. You could find that you have little time to mix with non-medics.
- While all the medical schools are well equipped and provide a high standard of teaching, there are real differences in the way the courses are taught and examined. Specifically, the majority offer an 'integrated course' in which students see patients at an early stage and certainly before the formal clinical part of the course. The other main distinction is between systems-based courses which teach medicine in terms of the

body's systems (eg the cardiovascular system) and subject-based courses which teach in terms of the fundamental subjects (anatomy, biochemistry, etc). The style of teaching can also vary from place to place. In particular, some medical schools use problem-based learning (PBL) extensively. For example, the course at East Anglia features PBL and the programme offers a variety of formats to encourage learning, including whole-class discussions, lectures, seminars and, especially, small-group sessions. Clinical, communication and IT skills are taught throughout. Within each year, clinical experience is provided in general practice and in hospitals. Assessment is on a unit-by-unit basis and includes: multiple-choice questionnaires; portfolios, presentations and projects; 'advanced notice' questions in which researched answers are presented under examination conditions and Objective Structured Clinical Examinations (OSCEs). These are matters of personal preference. You should consult the prospectus of each medical school in your own school's careers library. Once you have narrowed the choice down to about 10–12, it is worth writing to all those on your list for a copy of each prospectus. These will be sent to you free of charge.

■ Another difference in the courses offered concerns the opportunities for an intercalated Honours BSc and electives. The intercalated BSc scheme allows students to tack one further year of study either to the end of the two-year pre-clinical course, or as an integrated part of a six-year course. Successful completion of this year, which may be used to study a wide variety of subjects, confers a BSc degree qualification. Electives are periods of work experience away from the medical school and, in some cases, abroad.

■ Oxford and Cambridge are special cases. You can apply only to one and your teachers will tell you whether to apply to either. You would need a good reason to apply to Oxbridge against the advice of your teachers and it certainly is not worth applying on the 'off chance' of getting in. By doing so you will simply waste one of your valuable four choices.

WHAT THE SELECTOR LOOKS FOR

Most medical schools use a form which the selector fills in as he or she reads through your application. Have a look at the example opposite; below we go through the headings on this form.

MEDICAL INTERVIEW SELECTION FORM

Name	UCAS number
Age at entry	Gap year?
GCSE and AS results	AS/A-level predictions
Selector	Date

Selection Criteria	Areas of enquiry	Comments	Score (1–10)
Academic	1. GCSE results		
	2. A-level predictions		
Commitment	3. Genuine interest in medicine?		
	4. Relevant work experience?		
	5. Involvement in the community?		
Personal	6. Range of interests?		
	7. Involvement in school activities?		
	8. Evidence of achievements and/or leadership?		
	9. Does referee support application?		
		Total score	

Recommendation of selector	Call for interview	Score range 25–30
	Reserve list	Score range 16–24
	Rejection	Score range 0–15

Comments (if any)

Academic

1. GCSE: Points total and breadth of subjects

By the time you read this you will probably have chosen your GCSE subjects or even taken them. If you have not, here are some points to bear in mind:

- Medical school selectors like to see breadth. Try to take as many GCSE subjects as possible. Try to take at least eight but if your school places restrictions on the choice or number of GCSEs you take, make sure this fact is referred to in your confidential reference.
- You will almost certainly study two science/maths subjects at A-level and you will need to study chemistry. There is a big gap between GCSE and A-level. If you have the choice, don't make that jump even harder by studying combined or integrated science rather than the single science subjects. If your school will not allow you to study the single subjects, you should consider taking extra lessons during the summer holiday after your GCSE exams.
- Medical school selectors look at applicants' GCSE grades in considerable detail and some, such as St George's, actually use a points system, awarding three points for an A* or an A, two for a B, one for a C, and look for a minimum of 25 points over eight subjects; or 80 per cent at grade A for candidates not sitting eight subjects. Other schools adopt similar, if less formal, systems and most look for As in maths and the basic sciences. Many require a minimum of a B grade in English language. They hope to see As and Bs in the other subjects and will not be impressed by C grades and below. If you have yet to take GCSEs, work very hard to achieve these high grades. If you think you might do badly, consider taking extra lessons or an Easter revision course before the exam.
- If you have already taken your GCSEs and achieved disappointing grades, you must resign yourself to working exceptionally hard from the first day of your A-level course. You will also need to convince your UCAS referee that the GCSE grades are not an indicator of low grades at A-level, so that this can be mentioned in your reference.

2. AS-levels: Do they matter?

Under the old A-level system, the first year of the sixth form (year 12) could be a time for adjustment, contemplation and relaxation. Even if you studied modular A-levels, the marks did not feature on your UCAS form, and modules could be retaken again and again. The new system puts pressure on you from the start since not only do the grades appear on the form, but also many of the medical schools will specify minimum grade requirements. Even those that don't will consciously or subconsciously use them as an indicator or your likely A-level grades. Imagine the situation: the selector has one more interview slot to fill, and has the choice between two students with identical work experience, GCSE results and A-level predictions; but one has scored DDDD at AS-level, the other achieved AAAA. Who do you think will get the place? The other thing to bear in mind is that a score of DDDD is unlikely to lead to AAB at A-level since an AS contributes 50 per cent of the total A-level marks, and so the selectors may doubt that the predicted grades are achievable. You are probably aware of the fuss that surrounded the publication of the A-level results last year. One of the outcomes of the enquiry into the results was the growing awareness of the importance of retaking AS units if possible. Every extra mark gained on the (easier) AS units is a mark that you don't have to get in the (harder) A2 exams. If you have a second attempt at an AS unit, the board will take the higher of the two marks.

3. A-level predictions: Does your school expect at least ABB?

Your choice of A-levels
You will see from Table 1 that most medical schools now ask for just two science/maths subjects at A-level, with another science at AS-level. They all require chemistry and/or biology so you need to choose either physics or mathematics if you wish to apply to a medical school that requires three science subjects. There are three important considerations:

- Choose subjects that you are good at. You must be capable of an A grade. If you aren't sure, ask your teachers.
- Choose subjects that will help you in your medical course: life at medical school is tough enough as it is without having to learn new subjects from scratch.
- While it is acceptable to choose a non-scientific third AS or A-level which you enjoy and which will provide you with an interesting topic of conversation at your interview (and students who can cope with the differing demands of arts and sciences at A-level have an advantage in that they can demonstrate breadth), you should be careful not to choose subjects such as art which are practical rather than academic. General studies is not acceptable either.

What combination of subjects should you choose? In addition to chemistry and another science at A-level, you might also consider subjects such as psychology, business studies, sociology or a language at AS-level. The point to bear in mind when you are making your choices is that you need high grades, so do not pick a subject that sounds interesting, such as Italian, if you are not good at languages. Similarly, although an AS-level in statistics might look good on your UCAS form, you will not do well at it if you struggled at GCSE mathematics. You will need to check the individual requirements, but in general, it is likely that most medical schools will require at least one AS-level to be in an arts or humanities subject.

Taking four A-levels

There's no harm in doing more than three A-levels or four AS-levels, but you should drop the fourth/fifth subject if there is any danger of it pulling down your grades in the others. The medical schools will not include the fourth A-level in any conditional offers they make.

The prediction

The selector will look for a grade prediction in the reference that your headteacher writes about you. Your head will probably make a prediction based on the reports of your teachers, your GCSE grades and, most importantly, on the results of the school exams and AS-levels that you take at the end of your lower sixth-form year.

Consequently, it is vital that you work hard during the first year of A-levels. Only by doing so will you get the 'brownie points' you need. If there is any reason or excuse to explain why you did badly at GCSE or did not work hard in the lower sixth, you must make sure that the head knows about it and includes it in the reference. The most common reasons for poor performance are illness and problems at home (eg illness of a close relation or family breakdown).

The bottom line is that you need to persuade your head and your teachers that you are on line for grades of at least ABB. Convincing them usually involves convincing yourself!

Commitment

4. Have you shown a genuine interest in medicine?

This question has to be answered partly by your head in his or her reference and partly by you in section 10 of the UCAS form but, before we go on, it's time for a bit of soul-searching in the form of a short test, shown below. Get a piece of paper and do this immediately, before you read on.

The *Getting into Medical School* Genuine Interest Test

Instructions: Answer all the questions, truthfully.

1. Do you regularly read articles about medicine in:

    (a)   Daily (broadsheet) newspapers
    (b)   *New Scientist*
    (c)   *Student BMJ?*

2. Do you regularly watch Casualty, Holby City, ER or any medical documentaries such as How To Build a Human?

3. Do you possess any books or CD-ROMs about the human body or medicine, or do you visit medical web sites?

4. Have you attended a first-aid course?

5. Have you arranged a visit to your local GP?

6. Have you arranged to visit your local hospital in order to see the work of doctors at first hand?

7. What day of the week does your favourite newspaper publish a health section?

8. Do you know the main causes of death in this country?

9. Do you know what the following stand for:

    (a)   GMC
    (b)   BMA
    (c)   NICE
    (d)   AIDS
    (e)   BSE
    (f)   MS
    (g)   ECG?

Marking the test

You should have answered 'yes' to most of the first six questions and have been able to give answers to the last three. A low score (mainly 'No' and 'Don't know' answers) should make you ask yourself if you really are sufficiently interested in medicine as a career. If you achieved a high score, you need to ensure that you communicate your interest on the UCAS form. The next paragraphs explain how, but first a note about work experience and courses.

5. Have you had relevant work experience and courses?

In addition to the brief visits to your local hospital and GP's surgery (which you should be able to arrange through your school or with the help of your parents), it is important to undertake a longer period of relevant work experience. This will probably be unpaid but, when arranging this unpaid voluntary work, be choosy about the jobs you do. Don't accept routine clerical jobs or anything that doesn't bring you into contact with patients. Conversely, do accept work that involves the gritty, unglamorous side of patient care. A week spent helping elderly and confused patients walk to the toilet is worth a month in the hospital laboratory helping the technicians to carry out routine tests. Unfortunately, these hospital jobs are hard to get and you may have to offer to work at weekends or at night. If that fails, you should try your local hospice.

Hospices tend to be short of money because they are maintained by voluntary donations. They are usually happy to take on conscientious volunteers and the work they do (caring for the terminally ill) is particularly appropriate. Remember that you are not only working in a hospital/hospice in order to learn about medicine in action. You are also there to prove (to yourself as well as to the admissions tutors) that you have the dedication and stomach for what is often an unpleasant and upsetting work environment. You should be able to get the address of your nearest hospice from your GP's surgery.

When you come to write section 10 of your UCAS form you will want to describe your practical experience of medicine in some detail. Say what you did, what you saw and what insights you gained from it. As always, include details that could provide the signpost to an interesting question in your interview. For example, suppose you write:

During the year that I worked on Sunday evenings at St Sebastian's Hospice, I saw a number of patients who were suffering from cancer and it was interesting to observe the treatment they received and watch its effects.

A generous interviewer will ask you about the management of cancer and you have an opportunity to impress if you can explain the use of drugs, radiotherapy, diet, exercise, etc.

The other benefit of work in a medical environment is that you may be able to make a good impression on the senior staff you have worked for. If they are prepared to write a brief reference and send it to your head, he or she will be able to quote from it within the reference on the UCAS form.

Always keep a diary
During your work experience keep a diary and write down what you saw being done. At the time, you may think that you will remember what you saw, but there could be as long as 18 months between the work experience and an interview, and you will almost certainly forget vital details. Very often, applicants are asked at interview to talk more about something interesting on their UCAS form. For example:

Interviewer: *I see that you observed a coronary angioplasty. What does that involve?*

You: *Er.*

Interviewer: *Well, I know it's hard to see what's happening but I'm sure you understand the reason for carrying out a coronary angioplasty.*

You: *Um.*

Don't allow this to happen to you!

The only problem with work experience is that it can be hard to persuade members of a busy medical team to spend time explaining in detail what they are doing and why. MPW and a number of other organisations (see page 94) run courses for sixth-formers to help them understand the common areas of medicine and to link this theoretical knowledge to practical procedures.

6. Have you been involved in your local community?

A career in medicine involves serving the community and you need to demonstrate that you have something of the dedication needed to be a good doctor. You may have been able to do this through voluntary jobs in hospitals or hospices. If not, you need to think about devoting a regular period each week to one of the charitable organisations that care for those in need.

The number needing this help has increased following the government's decision to close some of the long-stay mental institutions and place the burden of caring for patients on local authorities. Your local social services department (address in the phone book) will be able to give you information on this and other opportunities for voluntary work. Again, it is helpful to obtain brief references from the people you work for so that these can be included in what your head writes about you.

Personal qualities

7. Have you demonstrated a range of interests?

Medical schools like to see applicants who have done more with their life than work for their A-levels and watch TV. While the head will probably refer to your outstanding achievements in his or her reference, you also need to say something about them in section 10. Selectors like to read about achievements in sport and other outdoor activities such as The Duke of Edinburgh's Award Scheme. Other useful activities include Young Enterprise, charity work, public speaking, part-time jobs, art, music and drama.

Bear in mind that selectors will be asking themselves, 'Would this person be an asset to the medical school?' Put in enough detail and try to make it interesting to read. Here is an example of a paragraph on interests for section 10.

I very much enjoy tennis and play in the school team and for Hampshire at under-18 level. This summer a local sports shop has sponsored me to attend a tennis camp in California. I worked at the Wimbledon championships in 2001.

I have been playing the piano since the age of eight and took my Grade 7 exams recently. At school, I play in the orchestra and in a very informal jazz band. Last year I started learning the trombone but I would not like anyone except my teacher to hear my playing!

I like dancing and social events but my main form of relaxation is gardening. I have started a small business helping my neighbours to improve their gardens – which also brings in some extra money!

And here's how not to do it:

I play tennis in competitions and the piano and trombone. I like gardening.

DIRE WARNINGS

1. Don't copy either of the paragraphs slavishly on to your own UCAS form.
2. Don't write anything that isn't true.
3. Don't write anything you can't talk about at the interview.
4. Avoid over-complicated, over-formal styles of writing. Read your personal statement out loud: if it doesn't sound like you speaking, rewrite it.

What if you aren't musical, can't play tennis and find geraniums boring? It depends when you are reading this. Anyone with enough drive to become a doctor can probably rustle up an interest or two in six months. If you haven't even got that long, then I suggest you devote most of section 10 to your interest in medicine.

8. Have you contributed to school activities?

This is largely covered by the section on interests but it is worth noting that the selector is looking for someone who will contribute to the communal life of the medical school. If you have been involved in organising things in your school do remember to include the details. If it's true, don't forget to say that you ran the school's fundraising barbecue or that you organised a sponsored jog in aid of handicapped children. Conversely, medical schools are less interested in applicants whose activities are exclusively solitary or which cannot take place in the medical school environment. Don't expect to get much credit for:

My main interest is going for long walks in desolate places by myself or in the company of my discman.

9. Have you any achievements to your credit?
Again, the main points have been covered already, but you should recall that the selectors are looking for applicants who stand out and who have done more with their lives than the absolute minimum. They are particularly attracted by excellence in any sphere. Have you competed in any activity at a high level or received a prize or other recognition for your achievements? If so, make sure that you include it in section 10.

10. To what extent does your referee support your application?
I have explained the vital importance of judicious grovelling to your referee and making sure that he or she knows all the good news about your work in hospitals and in the local community. Remember that the head will rely heavily on advice from other teachers too. They also need to be buttered up and helped to see you as a natural doctor. Come to school scrupulously clean and tidy. Work hard, look keen and make sure you talk about medicine in class. Ask intelligent, medicine-related questions such as:

'Is it because enzymes become denatured over 45°C that patients suffering from heat stroke have to be cooled down quickly using ice?'

or

'Could sex-linked diseases such as muscular dystrophy be avoided by screening the sperm to eliminate those containing the X chromosomes which carry the harmful recessive genes from an affected male?'

Your friends may find all this nauseating – ignore them. They'll be laughing on the other side of their faces when you're a doctor and they are still filling supermarket shelves.

If your referee is approachable you should be able to ask whether or not he or she feels able to support your application. In the unlikely case that he or she cannot recommend you, you should consider asking if another teacher could complete the form. This will look odd but even heads are human: clashes of personality do very occasionally occur and you must not let the medical schools receive a form which damns you.

THE MECHANICS OF THE UCAS FORM

You will receive advice from your school and you may also find it helpful to consult the MPW guide *How To Complete Your UCAS Form* (see page 96). Some additional points that apply chiefly to medicine are set out below.

Presentation: How your UCAS form looks

It is a well-known joke that doctors have dreadful handwriting. Sadly, that does not mean that you are allowed to write your life history in an illegible scrawl. If you can, use either the EAS (Electronic Application System) or the website version. These allow you to complete your UCAS form on a computer and to email it to UCAS. If your school does not offer EAS, try to make life easy for the selectors. Follow these tips:

- Make photocopies of the UCAS form and practise filling it in before you write on the real one.
- If you do make a mess of the real form, tear it up and ask your school for another one. You are entitled to use as many as you like providing that you submit only one to UCAS.
- Plan section 10 as you would plan an essay. Lay it out in a logical order. Make the sentences short and to the point. Split the section into paragraphs, with headings such as 'work experience', 'reasons for choice', 'interests' and 'achievements'. This will enable the selector to read and assess it quickly and easily.
- Don't write too much. Your form will be photocopied by UCAS and reduced to two-thirds of its original size. If you try to cram in too much and end up writing without paragraphs in a cramped and untidy style, the result will be illegible and selectors will give up before reaching the pearls you have cast before them.
- Construct section 10 on a word-processor and print or photocopy it onto the form. This overcomes problems of editing and illegibility. Selectors can still assess your handwriting from the other sections.

- Ask your parents, or someone else who is roughly the same age as the selectors (over 30), to cast a critical eye over your draft and don't be too proud to make changes in the light of their advice.

Timing: When to send in the form

The UCAS period is from 1 September to 15 January, but medical applications have to be with UCAS by 15 October. Late applications are also permitted, although the medical schools are not bound to consider them. Remember that most heads take at least a week to consult the relevant teachers and compile a reference, so allow for that and aim to hand in your form by 1 September unless there is a good reason for delaying.

The only convincing reason for delaying is that your teachers cannot predict high A-level grades at the moment but might be able to do so if they see high-quality work during the autumn term. If you are not on line for AAB/ABB by October, you still need to send in the form because, without an entry on the UCAS computer, you cannot participate in Clearing (see page 48).

 Keep a photocopy of your completed UCAS form so that you can look at it when you prepare for the interview

What happens next and what to do about it

When the staff at UCAS receive your form they send you the self-addressed card to show that it has arrived. If you don't receive this card within two weeks of handing in the form, you should check with your referee that it has been sent off. A few weeks later UCAS will send you a slip showing the details of your application. Check it carefully to make sure that the details you put on your form have been transferred correctly to the UCAS computer. At the same time make a note of your UCAS number – you will need to quote this when you contact the medical schools.

Now comes a period of waiting which can be very unsettling but which must not be allowed to distract you from your work. Most medical schools decide whether or not they want to interview you within a month but there are some categories, such as retake students, who will not be called for interview until the new year; in some cases, the medical school may wait until March when the results of any January retake exams are known.

If you have applied to one of those medical schools which do not interview, the next communication you receive may be a notification from UCAS that you have been made a conditional offer.

If one or more of the medical schools decides to interview you, your next letter will be an invitation to visit the school and attend an interview. (For advice on how to prepare for the interview see pages 22–43.)

If you are unlucky, the brown envelope from UCAS will contain the news that you have been rejected by one or more of your choices. Does that mean it's time to relax on the A-level work and dust off alternative plans? Should you be reading up exactly what the four-year course in 'Road Resurfacing' involves? No, you should not! A rejection is a setback and it does make the path into medicine that bit steeper, but it isn't an excuse to give up.

A rejection should act as a spur to work even harder because the grades you achieve at A-level are now more important. Don't give up and do turn to page 48 to see what to do when you get your A-level results.

SUCCEEDING IN THE INTERVIEW

The idea of preparing for an interview is a relatively new one, and there are still many people who feel that you can't (or shouldn't) do so. Nevertheless, there is a fundamental weakness in the theory that the panel will somehow dismiss what you say and how you look as they unerringly uncover the 'real you'. Wise and experienced the interviewers may be, but they do not have the ability to examine the deep recesses of the soul. They cannot ignore the words you didn't mean to say or supply the ones you left out.

Success in an interview, like success in any other human activity, depends on preparation and practice. The first time you try to do something you usually get it wrong, if only because unfamiliarity leads to nervousness. Practice is particularly important because the medical schools rarely give a second chance to someone who makes a bad impression at interview.

To help you practise, this chapter lists many typical questions and includes discussion of how to answer them. There is a section on how you can take charge of the interview and encourage the interviewers to ask you the questions you want to answer. Finally, there is a brief explanation of what will happen after your interviews.

The questions included here are real questions that have been put to applicants over the last two years. They have been gleaned from students who have faced interviews, admissions tutors, and through sitting in on the real thing. As explained later, one cannot prepare for the odd, unpredictable questions, but the interviewers are not trying to catch you out and they can be relied on to ask some of the general questions that are discussed here.

For many questions there are no 'right' answers and, even if there were, you shouldn't trot them out parrot fashion. The purpose of presenting the questions, and some strategies for answering them, is to help you think about your answers before the interview and to enable you to put forward your own views clearly and with confidence.

When you have read through this section, and thought about the questions, arrange for someone to sit down with you and take you through the mock interview questions in Appendix A on page 85. (If you have the facilities, you will find it helpful to record the interview on video, for later analysis.) You might be interested in the views of four medical professionals, quoted in the November 2002 edition of the *Student BMJ*, on the qualities that they look for;

Peter McCrorie, Director of the Graduate Entry Programme at St George's:

'... *an understanding about what being a good doctor entails from both the profession's point of view and the patient's point of view; a significant, meaningful experience of working in a healthcare environment or with disabled or disadvantaged people; an understanding of the importance of research in medicine; an awareness of the ethical issues associated with medical research; good oral communication skills and evidence of flexible and critical thinking.*'

Dr Allan Cumming, Associate Dean of Teaching at Edinburgh University:

'*The innate characteristics of a good doctor are beneficence and the capacity to engage with the knowledge necessary for informed practice.*'

Mike Shooter, President of the Royal College of Psychiatrists:

'*I think that you are born with some personal qualities, such as the ability to get on with people, to empathise with their distress, to inspire confidence in others, and to carry anxiety. Such qualities are very difficult to train into a person. A good doctor also needs knowledge and the experience of implementing that knowledge.*'

John Tooke, Dean of the Peninsula Medical School:

'*A medical student needs to be bright – not least to cope with a lifetime of assimilation of new concepts and knowledge. The ability to communicate, the ability to work as part of a multi-professional team, empathy and a non-prejudicial approach are qualities that should be expected in all healthcare professionals. There is also, however, a need for diversity and a need to resist any move towards personality conformity.*'

Finally, don't forget that medical school interviewers are busy people and they do not interview for the fun of it. Neither do they set out to trip you up or humiliate you. They call you for interview because they want to offer you a place – make it easy for them to do so!

TYPICAL INTERVIEW QUESTIONS AND HOW TO TACKLE THEM

Questions designed to test motivation

1. 'Why do you want to become a doctor?'
The question that most interviewees dread! Answers that will turn your interviewers' stomachs and may lead to rejection are:

'I want to heal sick people.'

'My father is a doctor and I want to be like him.'

'The money's good and unemployment among doctors is low.'

'The careers teacher told me to apply.'

'It's glamorous.'

'I want to join a respected profession, so it is either this or Law.'

Try the question now. Most sixth-formers find it quite hard to give an answer and are often not sure why they want to be a doctor. Often the reasons are lost in the mists of time and have simply been reinforced over the years.

The interviewers will be sympathetic but they do require an answer that sounds convincing. There are four general strategies:

1. The story (Option A)
You tell the interesting (and true) story of how you have always been interested in medicine, how you have made an effort to find out what is involved by visiting your local hospital, working with your GP, etc and how this long-term and deep-seated interest has now become something of a passion. (Stand by for searching questions designed to check that you know what you are talking about!)

2. The story (Option B)

You tell the interesting (and true) story of how you, or a close relative, suffered from an illness which brought you into contact with the medical profession. This experience made you think of becoming a doctor and, since then, you have made an effort to find out what is involved ... (as before).

3. The logical elimination of alternatives

In this approach you have analysed your career options and decided that you want to spend your life in a scientific environment (you have enjoyed science at school) but would find pure research too impersonal. Therefore the idea of a career that combines the excitement of scientific investigation with a great deal of human contact is attractive. Since discovering that medicine offers this combination you have investigated it (and other alternatives) thoroughly (visits to hospitals, GPs, etc) and have become passionately committed to your decision.

The problems with this approach are that:

- they will have heard it all before
- you will find it harder to convince them of your passion for medicine.

4. Fascination with people

Some applicants can honestly claim to have a real interest in people. Here's a test to see if you are one:

You are waiting in the queue for a bus/train/supermarket checkout, etc. Do you ignore the other people in the queue or do you start chatting to them? Win extra points if they spontaneously start chatting to you and a bonus if, within five minutes, they have told you their life story. Applicants with this magical power to empathise with their fellow human beings do, if they have a matching interest in human biology, have a good claim to a place at medical school.

Whether you choose one of these strategies or one of your own, your answer must be well considered and convincing. Additionally, it should sound natural and not over-rehearsed. Bear in mind that most of your interviewers will be doctors, and they will have (hopefully) chosen medicine because they, like you, had a burning desire to do so. They will not expect you to be able to justify your choice by reasoned argument alone. Statements (as long as they are supported by evidence of practical research) such as '... *and the more work I did at St James's, the more I realised that*

medicine is what I desperately want to do ...' are quite acceptable – and far more convincing than saying '*Medicine is the only career that combines science and the chance to work with people*' because it isn't!

2. 'What have you done to show your commitment to medicine and to the community?'

This should tie in with your UCAS form. Your answer should demonstrate that you do have a genuine interest in helping others. Ideally, you will have a track record of regular visits to your local hospital or hospice where you will have worked on the less attractive side of patient care (such as cleaning bedpans). Acceptable alternatives are regular visits to an elderly person to do their chores, or work with one of the charities that care for the homeless or other distressed groups.

It isn't sufficient to have worked in a laboratory, out of sight of patients, or to have done so little work as to be trivial. ('*I once walked around the ward of the local hospital – it was very nice.*')

You may find this leads the interviewer to ask: '*If you enjoyed working in the hospital so much, why don't you want to become a nurse?*' This is a tough question. You need to indicate that, while you admire enormously the work that nurses do, you would like the challenge of diagnosis and of deciding what treatment should be given.

3. 'Why have you applied to this medical school?'

Don't say:

'*It's well equipped*'

'*I like the buildings*'

'*It's easy to get into*'

'*My dad's the Dean*'

'*It has a good reputation*' (unless you know exactly what for).

Some of the reasons that you might have are:

■ You have made a thorough investigation of a number of the medical schools that you have considered. You have been to an open day and talked to current medical students. You have spoken to the admissions tutor about your particular situation, and to ask their advice about

suitable work experience, and he or she was particularly encouraging and helpful. You feel that the general atmosphere is one you would love to be part of.

■ You have read the prospectus (don't forget to) and feel that the course is structured in an interesting way. You like the fact that it is integrated and that students are brought into contact with patients at an early date. Another related reason might be that you are attracted by the subject-based or system-based teaching approach. A subject-based course covers the material in terms of academic subjects like biochemistry or anatomy whereas a systems-based course looks at the body's systems (eg the cardiovascular system).

■ Your careers teacher at school recommended the school. Careers teachers make it their business to find out about individual medical schools and they will also receive feedback from their former pupils. An informed recommendation is a perfectly valid reason for choosing a particular medical school. The same applies to advice you may read in this or other books.

■ A variation on the careers teacher theme: you may have a recommendation from your own personal friends or informed friends of your parents. In this case you must be able to quote the names of these friends.

■ Don't forget that all the UK medical schools and university departments of medicine are well equipped and offer a high standard of teaching. It is therefore perfectly reasonable to say that, while you have no specific preference at this stage, you do have a great deal to give to any school that offers you a place. This answer will, inevitably, lead on to: '*Well, tell us what you do have to give?*' That question is discussed on page 38.

Questions designed to assess your knowledge of medicine

No one expects you to know all about your future career before you start at medical school, but they do expect you to have made an effort to find out something about it. If you are really interested in medicine, you will have a reasonable idea of common illnesses and diseases, and you will be aware of topical issues. Remember the 'Genuine Interest Test' on page 13. The questions divide into six main areas:

1. The human body (and what can go wrong with it)

The interviewers will expect you to be interested in medicine and to be aware of current problems and new treatments. In both cases the list is endless but the following are some areas with which you should familiarise yourself.

Your personal area of interest
This is how the questions might go.

Interviewer: *You have written on your UCAS form that you are interested in how the human body works. Which system particularly interests you?*
You: *Um, the brain.*
Interviewer: *Tell us how the brain works.*
You: *Um, oh dear. I'm very sorry, I've forgotten.*
Interviewer: *(with pleasure as they spring the trap) Well, that's a real pity because there are only two people in the world who know how the brain works. One is God and he won't tell us and the other is you and you've forgotten. (Laughs all round at your expense.)*

Avoid this trap by choosing, in advance, a relatively well-understood body system such as the cardiovascular system, then learn how it works and (particularly for interviews at Oxbridge) prepare for fundamental questions like:

'What is meant by myocardial infarction?'

and questions about what can go wrong with the system – see below.

Your own work experience
If you are able to arrange work experience in a medical environment you will want to include it in section 10 of your UCAS form but make sure that you keep a diary and that you enter in it not only what you saw but medical details of what was happening. For example, note not only that a patient was brought into casualty but what the symptoms were, what the diagnosis was and what treatment was given.

A Point to Note: Interviewers are looking for a genuine enthusiasm for medicine. They are not going to be impressed by a long list of hospital departments' treatments or illnesses unless they can see that your experience actually meant something to you on a personal level, and that you gained insights into the profession.

An example of a bad answer
Interviewer: *I notice that you spent two weeks at St James's. Tell me something about what you did there.*
You: *I spent two days in the Cardiology department, three days in A&E, one day in the Pathology lab, two days in an Oncology ward, one and a half days in Neurology and half a day in General Surgical. I saw sutures, drips, lung cancer ... [etc]*

The problem here is that the interviewers are no clearer about your suitability for a career in medicine, only that you have a good memory. This is referred to by some admissions tutors as 'medical tourism'.

A better answer
You: *I was able to spend time in a number of wards, which enabled me to see a whole range of treatments. For instance, during my two days in the Cardiology department, I was able to see several newly admitted patients who might have had heart attacks. I found it particularly interesting to see how careful the doctors had to be in taking the history, so that they were not putting words into the patients' mouths about their symptoms, and the type of pain they were experiencing. I was also able to watch an angioplasty being performed. I was amazed at the level of skill the surgeon demonstrated – I would love to do that myself one day.*

In this type of answer, your genuine enthusiasm, good observation and respect for the profession are all apparent.

Keeping a file of cuttings
Make sure that you read *New Scientist*, *Student BMJ* and, on a daily basis, a broadsheet newspaper which carries regular, high-quality medical reporting. *The Independent* has excellent coverage of current health issues, and the *Guardian's* health section on Tuesdays is informative and interesting. The Sunday broadsheets often contain comprehensive summaries of the week's top medical stories.

The big killers
Diseases affecting the circulation of the blood (including heart disease) and cancer are the main causes of death in the UK. Make sure you know

the factors that contribute towards them and the strategies for prevention and treatment. Their importance is illustrated by the following table.

Selected causes of death in the UK for 1999
(to nearest 1,000)

Cause of death	Total deaths 1999	Total deaths 1996
Cancer (total)	150,000 (52% men)	156,000
Lung cancer	34,000 (62% men)	36,000
Breast cancer (women)	13,000	14,000
Prostate cancer (men)	9,000	10,000
Circulatory diseases (including heart)	250,000 (52% women)	270,000
Myocardial infarction + Ischaemic heart disease	132,000 (55% men)	148,000
Cerebrovascular	65,000 (63% women)	68,000
Pneumonia	66,000 (61% women)	66,000
Accidents (all)	13,000	12,000
Traffic accidents	3,000	4,000
Total deaths in UK	**630,000**	**635,000**

Source: World Health Organisation

You should be able to discuss possible reasons for the changes in death rates from causes such as cancer and heart problems, and for the difference in mortality rates between men and women.

The global picture

The world population is about 6 billion, and growing. Last year, around 60 million people died. The biggest killers are infectious diseases (13 million) such as AIDS, malaria and tuberculosis; and circulatory diseases (17 million) such as coronary heart disease and stroke. Cancer killed about 7 million people.

Infectious diseases that were once thought to be under control, such as tuberculosis, cholera and yellow fever, have made comebacks. This is due, in part, to the increasing resistance of certain bacteria to antibiotics. The antibiotics that we use now are essentially modifications to drugs that have been in use for the last 30 or 40 years, and random genetic mutations allow resistant strains to multiply. Current Issues (page 60) gives more background information, including an assessment of the differences between developed and developing countries' health issues.

The effects of an ageing population

Life expectancy continues to rise (except in many sub-Saharan African countries which have been ravaged by HIV/AIDS – see page 78) because of improvement in sanitation and medical care. Birth rates in most countries are falling, and the combination of the two brings considerable problems. The relative numbers of people who succumb to chronic illness (such as cancer, diabetes, cataract, diseases of the circulatory system) is increasing and this puts greater strains on countries' health care systems. A useful indicator is the Dependency Ratio – the percentage of the population that is economically dependent on the active age group. It is calculated as the sum of 0–14-year-olds and over-65-year-olds, divided by the number of people aged between 15 and 59. This is rising steadily. The World Health Organisation's website contains data for each country. The address can be found at the end of the book.

The Human Genome Project and gene therapy

Arguably, the most important scientific work of the last century was the discovery of the structure of DNA and the identification of the human genes. The Human Genome Project, the mapping of all human genes, made great progress during the 1990s and many of the illnesses that have their origins in genetic defects were identified. The defective genes have been listed and tests developed to enable the individuals who carry them to be made aware of the fact. This in itself raises some ethical and moral issues.

You would be wise to familiarise yourself with the sequence of developments in the field of genetic research, starting with the discovery of the double helix structure of DNA by Crick and Watson in 1953. You should find out all that you can about:

- Recombinant DNA technology (gene therapy, genetic engineering)
- Genetic diagnosis (of particular interest to insurance companies)
- Cloning (see page 73)
- Stem cell research
- GM crops
- Genetic enhancement of food animals
- 'Pharming'.

Fashionable illnesses

At any one time the media tend to concentrate on one or two 'fashionable' diseases. The papers fill their pages with news of the latest 'epidemic' and the general public is expected to react as if the great plague of 1665 were just round the corner. In reality, ebola and Creutzfeldt-Jakob disease (CJD) result in very small numbers of deaths. The media encourage us to react emotionally rather than logically in matters concerning risk. They advise us to stop eating beef but not to stop driving our cars even though around 3000 people were killed in road accidents in 1999.

While these diseases tend to be trivial in terms of their effect, they are often interesting in scientific terms and the fact that they are being discussed in the media makes it likely that they will come up at interview. A typical question would be:

'What is thought to be the infecting agent that causes CJD?'
It is important to know something about these illnesses (see Current Issues, page 69, for a discussion of mad cows and CJD) but equally important to keep them in statistical proportion.

Diet, exercise and the environment

The maintenance of health on a national scale isn't simply a matter of waiting until people get ill and then rushing in with surgery or medicine to cure them. There is good evidence that illness can be prevented by sensible diet, not smoking, taking exercise and living in a healthy environment. In this context, a healthy environment means one where food and water are uncontaminated by bacteria and living quarters are well ventilated, warm and dry. The huge advance in health and life expectancy since the middle of the nineteenth century owes much more to these factors than to the achievements of modern medicine.

A note on terminology

When discussing medical topics you will sound more convincing if you learn and use the correct terminology. For example, to a doctor, a patient doesn't turn up at the surgery with high blood pressure, he presents with hypertension. The best source of the correct terminology is medical textbooks, some of which are quite easy to understand (see Appendix D on page 94).

2. The medical profession

The typical question is: *'What makes a good doctor?'* Avoid answering: *'A caring and sympathetic nature.'* If these really were the crucial qualities of a good doctor there would be little point in going to medical school. Start by stressing the importance of the aspects that can be taught and, in particular, emphasise the technical qualities that a doctor needs: the ability to carry out a thorough examination, to diagnose accurately and quickly what is wrong and the skill to choose and organise the correct treatment.

After this comes the ability to communicate effectively and sympathetically with the patient so that he or she can understand and participate in the treatment. The most important part of communication is listening. There is an old medical adage that if you listen to the patient for long enough he or she will give you the diagnosis.

Communications skills also have an important role to play in treatment – studies have shown that some patients get better more quickly when they feel involved and part of the medical team. If you want, you can conclude with: *'good personal organisation and stamina for the famous 80-hour week.'*

3. The National Health Service – funding health

An application to a medical school is also an application for a job and you should have taken the trouble to find out something about your likely future employer. The questions *'Is there anything wrong with the NHS?'* and *'What would you do if you were the Secretary of State for Health?'* are tricky. Your first move should be to recognise and state that the core of the NHS consists, for the most part, of highly dedicated people working extremely hard and that the vast majority of patients speak very highly of the treatment they have received.

So what is wrong? The main problems of the NHS centre on the long waiting lists for treatment and the long hours worked by doctors. In the end, both come down to money – or the lack of it. The Conservative government believed that the old, pre-1992, structure of the service did not allow efficient use of resources. Hence its reforms of which you must be aware (see Current Issues, page 60). These reforms were unpopular with some sections of the medical profession, the criticism being that they put 'profits before patients'. In December 1997, the new Labour government published a White Paper: The New NHS; a summary of the

33

recommendations for modernisation that it contains, and the developments that followed, are in Current Issues (page 60).

Consider this line of questioning:

Interviewer: *If you were in charge, would you spend more money on the NHS?*
You: *Yes.*
Interviewer: *Where would you get the money from?*

It's best not to go down this path which, in essence, leads to a discussion of economics and politics rather than medicine. If you do get trapped, you should show that you know the facts. You could then list the five main sources of extra money:

1. Higher taxes.
2. Increased use of private health insurance (another form of tax).
3. More government borrowing.
4. Reallocation of money from other government programmes.
5. Change the balance of spending so that less is spent on administration and more is spent on treatment.

Historically, no government has found it possible to give the NHS all the money it needs when the costs of drugs and new equipment are rising much faster than inflation. One must conclude that full funding for the NHS, which would be a great vote winner at any election, is very difficult. If the finest political and economic brains in the country have failed to find a solution, you probably won't either.

4. Private medicine
Another set of questions that needs careful thought concerns private medicine. Don't forget that many consultants have flourishing private practices and rely on private work for a major part of their income. Equally, a number of doctors do not have the opportunity to practise privately and may resent a system that allows some consultants to earn money both within and outside the NHS.

Your best bet is to look at the philosophy behind private medicine and you may care to argue as follows:

'Most people agree that if you are run over by a bus you should be taken to hospital and treated at the taxpayers' expense. In general, urgent

treatment for serious and life-threatening conditions should be treated by the NHS and we should all chip in to pay for it. On the other hand, most of us would agree that someone who doesn't particularly care for the shape of his nose and who wants to change it by expensive plastic surgery should pay for the operation himself. We can't ban cosmetic operations so we are led to accept the right of private medicine to exist.'

Having established these two extremes, one is left to argue about the point where the two systems meet. Should there be a firm dividing line or a fuzzy one where both the NHS and private medicine operate? Currently the line is fuzzy.

You could also point out that private medicine should not harm the NHS. For example, the NHS has a problem of waiting lists. If ten people are standing in a queue for a bus, everyone benefits if four of those waiting jump into a taxi. Providing, of course, that they don't persuade the bus driver to drive it!

Now try this question yourself: 'Is it fair that a rich person should be able to buy better health than a poor person?' (Hint: start by examining the assumption made in the question.)

 TIP   This question illustrates an effective general technique for answering difficult moral, ethical or legal questions. The interviewers are not particularly interested in your opinion, but they are interested in whether you have understood the issues. Always demonstrate this by explaining the extreme opposing views. Only then, and in a balanced and reasonable way, give your own opinion.

5. Ethical questions
Medical ethics is a fascinating area of moral philosophy. You won't be expected to answer questions on the finer points but you could be asked about the following.

Abortion
Whatever your religious views, you need to know the law. Abortions cannot be performed after the 28th week (24th in practice) unless the mother's life is threatened, or there is evidence of foetal abnormality. Abortions are only legal on certain grounds, including:

- continuation of the pregnancy would cause permanent injury (mental or physical) to the mother

35

- the substantial risk that the child would be severely mentally or physically handicapped
- the woman's other children's health could be at risk.

To be legal, the abortion needs to be certified by two doctors.

You must also be prepared for the panel to present a scenario in which you would not be happy to perform an abortion. For example, a woman from an ethnic minority has learned as a result of amniocentesis that she is carrying a female child. Girls are of no value in her culture and, against her wishes, her husband insists she has an abortion. If a woman asks for an abortion which you could not carry out you must not try to dissuade her. You should refer her to another doctor who might be prepared to perform the operation.

Operations against the patient's will
This heading covers all action taken to preserve life when the patient or parent of the patient refuses to permit treatment. A classic case is the fundamentalist Christian who refuses a life-saving blood transfusion because it contravenes his or her religious beliefs. Fair enough, you may feel, but what if, on these grounds, a parent refuses to allow a baby's life to be saved by a transfusion? Similarly, in a well-publicised legal case, a woman refused to allow a Caesarean delivery of her baby. The judge ruled that the wishes of the mother could be overruled. It is worth noting that the NHS (as a representative of the state) has no right to keep a patient in hospital against his or her will unless the medical team and relatives use the powers of the Mental Health Act.

Euthanasia
Start by making sure that you know the law: mercy killing, in the sense of administering drugs to kill a patient who is in great pain, is illegal in this country – it is not in Holland. What is not illegal, and happens every day, is that life-supporting treatment is withdrawn and the patient dies from natural causes. You should also be aware of the difference between euthanasia (where a doctor or another person actively terminates a person's life) and physician-assisted suicide (where the doctor provides the patient with the means to commit suicide), and of the fact that many doctors see a moral distinction between the two. You should find out about the case of Diane Pretty.

The question is '*Could you withdraw treatment from a patient for whom the prognosis was very poor, who seemed to enjoy no quality of life and who was in great pain?*'

The answer to this question comes in two parts. First, you must recognise that a decision like this could not be taken without the benefit of full medical training and some experience, together with the advice of colleagues and the fullest consultation with the patient and his or her relations. If, after that process, it was clear that life support should be withdrawn, then, and only then, would you take your decision. Part two involves convincing the panel that, having taken your decision, you would act on it.

Difficult choices – who should be treated at public expense?
A good opening question is '*Should smokers be treated on the NHS?*' On the one hand, one can argue that all citizens and certainly all taxpayers have the right to treatment irrespective of their lifestyles. Conversely, it is certainly true that smoking is a contributory factor in heart disease. Is it fair to expect the community as a whole to spend a great deal of money on, for example, coronary artery bypass surgery if the patient refuses to abandon behaviour that could jeopardise the long-term effectiveness of the operation?

Another series of questions recognises the fact that there is a limit to the resources available to the NHS and highlights the tough decisions that may need to be taken. The questioner might refer to 'rationing of healthcare' (see Appendix A on page 85). Suppose you have resources for one operation but two critically ill patients – how do you decide which one to save? Or, suppose that you can perform six hip replacement operations for the cost of one coronary artery bypass. Heart bypass operations save life; hip replacements merely improve it. Which option should you go for?

Even more controversial issues surround surgery to change gender. Should these operations be performed when the money could be used to save, or least to prolong, life?

6. Other issues
Events are constantly bringing fresh moral issues associated with medicine into the public arena. It is important that you read the papers and maintain an awareness of the current 'hot' issues. See Appendix D (page 94) for further reading.

Questions aimed at finding out if you will fit in

One of the reasons for interviewing you is to see whether you will fit successfully in to both medical school and the medical profession. The interviewers will try to find out if your views and approach to life are likely to make you an acceptable colleague in a profession which, to a great extent, depends on teamwork. This does not mean that they want to hear views identical to their own. On the contrary, they will welcome ideas that are refreshing and interesting. What they do not like to hear is arrogance, lies, bigotry or tabloid headlines.

These questions have another important purpose: to assess your ability to communicate in a friendly and effective way with strangers even when under pressure. This skill will be very important when you come to deal with patients.

Questions about your UCAS form

Section 10, the section in which you write about yourself, is a fertile area for questions and, as explained earlier, you should have included some juicy morsels to attract the interviewers. The most successful interviews often revolve around some interesting or amusing topic that is fun to talk about and which makes you stand out from the crowd. The trouble is that you cannot invent such a topic – it really has to exist. Nevertheless, if you really have been involved in a campaign to save an obscure species of toad and can tell a couple of amusing stories about it (make them short), so much the better.

Even if your UCAS form seems, in retrospect, a bit dull, don't worry. Work out something interesting to say. Look at the photocopy of your form and at all costs avoid the really major disasters: if you wrote that you like reading, for instance, make sure you can remember and talk intelligently about the last book you read.

Sometimes an amusing comment on your form followed up by a relaxed and articulate performance at the interview will do the trick. A good example is the comment that a student made about lasting only three days as a waitress during the summer holidays. She was able to tell a story about dropped food and dry-cleaning bills, and was offered a place.

Questions about your contribution to the life of the medical school

These questions can come in many forms but, once identified, they need to be tackled carefully. If you say you like social life, they will worry that you won't pass your pre-clinical exams. If you say that you plan to spend your time windsurfing, mountaineering or fishing, they'll see you as a loner.

Probably the best approach is to say that you realise that medical school is hard work and that your main responsibility must be to pass your exams. After that, you could say that the medical school can only function as a community if the individuals involved are prepared to participate enthusiastically in as many of the extracurricular activities as possible. Above all, try to talk about communal and team activities rather than the more solitary pursuits.

You may find it helpful to know that, in one London medical school, the interviewers are told to ask themselves if the candidate has made good use of the opportunities available to them, and whether they have the personal qualities and interests appropriate to student life and a subsequent career in medicine. Poor communication skills, excessive shyness or lack of enthusiasm concern them, and will be taken into account when awarding scores.

Unpredictable questions

There are two types of unpredictable questions: nice and nasty.

Nice questions

Nice questions are usually designed to test your communication skills and to assess your personality. A typical nice question would be *'If you won a million pounds on the lottery, what would you do with it?'*

Rule 1: Don't relax! Your answer to this question needs to be as effective and articulate as any other and, while you should appear to be relaxed, you must not let your thinking or speech become sloppy.

Rule 2: A nice question could also indicate that the interviewer has decided against you and simply wants to get through the allotted time as easily as possible. If you suspect that this is the case (possibly because you have said something that you now regret), this question provides an opportunity to redeem yourself. Try to steer the questions back to gritty, medically related topics. See the advice on page 42.

Nasty questions

The 'interview nasties' are included either as a test of your reaction to pressure or in response to something you have said in answer to a previous question. Here are some examples:

'Why should we give you a place here when we have many better qualified applicants?'

'Don't you think that someone with the views you have just expressed would find it almost impossible to function effectively as an NHS doctor?'

There are no right answers but there is a correct approach. Start by fixing the questioner a big smile then distance the question from your own case. Taking the first question, you could say that you realise that medical school selection is a tough business and that the criteria must be hard to define. On the one hand it must be tempting to select those whose previous work indicates that they will sail through their pre-clinical exams but, on the other, you can think of brilliant academics who find it hard to communicate. You believe that you do have something to offer the profession.

In general, the technique once again is to identify the extreme answers to the question and then, almost as an afterthought, give your own position. This approach shows the interviewers that you are capable of logical reasoning under pressure.

Questions about your own academic performance

These are especially likely if you are retaking A-levels (or have retaken them). The question will be *'Why did you do so badly in your A-levels?'* Don't say *'I'm thick and lazy'* however true you feel that is!

Another bad ploy is to blame your teachers. It's part of the unspoken freemasonry of teaching that no teacher likes to hear another teacher blamed for poor results. If, however, your teacher was absent for part of the course, it is perfectly acceptable to explain this. You should also explain any other external circumstances such as illness or family problems even if you believe them to have been included in the UCAS reference. Sadly, most applicants don't have one of these cast-iron excuses!

The best answer, if you can put your hand on your heart when you deliver it, is to say that you were so involved in other school activities (head of school, captain of cricket, rowing and athletics, chairman of the Community Action Group and producer of the school play) that your work suffered. You can't really be blamed for getting the balance between work and your other activities a little bit skewed and even if you don't have a really impressive list of other achievements you should be able to construct an answer on this basis. You might also add that the setback allowed you to analyse your time management skills, and that you now feel you are much more effective in your use of time.

You may also be asked how you expect to do in your A-level exams. You need to show that you are working hard, enjoying the subjects and expect to achieve at least ABB (or more probably AAB – check Table 1 on page 81 for admissions policies to the different medical schools).

Your questions for the interviewers

At the end of the interview the person chairing the panel may ask if you have any questions you would like to put to the interviewers. Bear in mind that the interviews are carefully timed, and that your attempts to impress the panel with 'clever' questions may do quite the opposite. The golden rule is: only ask a question if you are genuinely interested in the answer (and which, of course, you were unable to find during your careful reading of the prospectus).

Questions to avoid are:

What is the structure of the first year of the course?

Will I be able to live in a hall of residence?

When will I first have contact with patients?

Can you tell me about the intercalated BSc option?

As well as being boring questions, the answers to these will be available in the prospectus. You have obviously not done any serious research.

Questions you could ask:

I haven't studied physics A-level. Do you think I should go through some physics textbooks before the start of the course?

This shows that you are keen, and that you want to make sure that you can cope with the course. It will give them a chance to talk about the extra course they offer for non-physicists.

Do you think I should try to get more work experience before the start of the course?

Again, an indication of your keenness.

Earlier, I couldn't answer the question you asked me on why smoking causes coronary heart disease. What is the reason?

Something that you genuinely might want to know.

How soon will you let me know if I have been successful or not?

Something you really want to know.

Remember: if in doubt, don't ask a question. End by saying *'All of my questions have been answered by the prospectus and the students who showed me around the medical school. Thank you very much for an enjoyable day.'* Big smile, shake hands and say goodbye.

HOW TO STRUCTURE THE INTERVIEW TO YOUR ADVANTAGE

Having read this far you may well be asking yourself what to do if none of the questions discussed come up. Some of them will. Furthermore, once the interviewers have asked one of the prepared questions, you should be able to lead them on to the others. This technique is very simple and most interviewers are prepared to go along with it because it makes their job easier. All you have to do is insert a 'signpost' at the end of each answer.

Let me give you an example. At the end of your answer to why you want to be a doctor you could add: *'I realise, of course, that medicine is moving through a period of exciting challenges and advances.'* Now stop and give the questioner an 'Over to you – I'm ready for the next question' look. Unless he or she is really trying to throw you off balance, the next question will be *'What do you know about these advances?'* Off you go with your answer but at the end you tack on: *'Hand in hand with these technical changes have come changes in the administration of the NHS.'* With luck, you'll get a question about the NHS which you can answer and end with a 'signpost' to medical ethics.

You can, if you wish, plan the whole interview so that each answer leads to a new question. The last answer can be linked to the first question so as to form a loop. The interviewers have only to ask one of the questions in the loop and you are off on a pre-planned track. This idea never works perfectly but it does enable you to maximise the amount of time you spend on prepared ground, time when, with luck, you'll be making a good impression. The disadvantage, of course, in having a set of preprepared answers ready is that there is a temptation to pull one out of the hat regardless of what is actually being asked. The question *'Why do you want to be a doctor?'* (which you might be expecting) requires a very different answer to the question *'Was there something that started your interest in being a doctor?'*

One final piece of advice on interviews: keep your answers short. Nothing is more depressing than an answer that rambles on. If you get a question you haven't prepared, pause for thought, give them your best shot in a cheerful, positive voice and then shut up.

WHAT HAPPENS NEXT

When you have left the room the person chairing the interview panel will discuss your performance with the other members and will make a recommendation to the Dean. The recommendation will be one of the following:

- Accept
- Discuss further/waiting list
- Reject.

Accept means that you will receive a conditional or unconditional offer, usually the standard one (see Table 1, page 81).

Discuss further means that you are borderline and may or may not receive an offer depending on the quality of the applicants seen by other interview panels. If, having been classified as 'Discuss further', you are unlucky and receive a rejection, the medical school may put you on an official or unofficial waiting list. The people on the waiting list are the first to be considered in Clearing. In 2003, UCAS has introduced an extra scheme, UCAS Extra, which allows applicants who have been rejected by all of the institutions to which they applied a chance to approach other universities. Details can be found on the UCAS website.

Reject means that you have not been made an offer. You may be luckier at one of the other medical schools to which you have applied, or you may have to wait and try to obtain a place through Clearing.

The official notification of your fate will come to you from UCAS within a few weeks of the interview. If you have been rejected it is helpful to know if you are on the waiting list and whether or not there is any point in applying again to that medical school. Understandably, the staff will be reluctant to talk to you about your performance but most medical schools will discuss your application with your UCAS referee if he or she rings them to ask what advice should now be given to you. It is well worth asking your head to make that telephone call.

GETTING THE RIGHT A-LEVEL GRADES

This isn't a study skills text and a full explanation of how to achieve high A-level grades is beyond the scope of this guide. Nevertheless, it is important that you know:

- What grades you require
- How to check if you are on line for them
- The factors that go to make up a good A-level grade.

These points are covered and, in addition, some specific advice on revision technique is included because this is an area which so often leads to difficulties. Finally, we give advice on what to do if things go wrong during the exams themselves.

THE GRADES YOU REQUIRE

Table 1 (page 81) shows that, with few exceptions, the grades you need for medicine are AAB. You might be lucky and get an offer of ABB but you will not know that until six months before the exams and you can't rely on it. As a general guide, students who have studied the IB are likely to need around 35 points, including 665 at Higher Level (including Chemistry); candidates who have studied under the Scottish system will need ABB in CSYS or Advanced Highers; and European Baccalaureate students will need a minimum of about 75 per cent overall, with at least 80 per cent in chemistry and another Full Option science/mathematical subject.

HOW TO ASSESS YOUR PROGRESS

For many A-level science subjects the A grade starts at between 72 per cent and 75 per cent so, to be sure of hitting your target (or exceeding it), you must ensure that you are hitting the high 70s in tests and mock exams. For exams in maths, or in modular papers, the A grade may start at a higher percentage.

FACTORS CONTRIBUTING TO GOOD EXAM RESULTS

If your mock exam or test results indicate that you are falling below A grade standard, the reasons may not be hard to find and rectify. Most A-level students know what they are doing wrong and, even if they don't, their teachers are usually only too glad to enlighten them.

WARNING: Do not allow good marks in homework to lull you into a false sense of security. Homework is important but what really counts in assessing progress is your performance in tests and mock exams. To be a valid predictor, the test must consist of real exam questions attempted under exam conditions in the time allowed for the real thing. Equally important is the marking of these tests which must follow the same approach as that employed by the examiners. For guidance on this you can consult the examiners' reports published by the examination boards.

HOW TO REVISE

Revision is what turns hard work into high grades. It is of crucial importance but often undertaken in a hurried, unplanned and ineffective manner. Good (that is, active – not simply reading notes) revision can so easily make the difference of the 5–10 per cent which can lift your exam result from a high C to an A.

Appendix C on page 91 gives some revision advice for A-level students as they begin their final revision period. Arguably, that is too late. To be really effective, revision needs to be a continuous process running in parallel with your coverage of the syllabus.

WHAT TO DO IF THINGS GO WRONG DURING THE EXAMS

If something happens when you are preparing for or actually taking the exams which prevents you from doing your best, you must notify both the exam board and the medical schools that have made you offers. This notification will come best from your headteacher and should include your UCAS number. Send it off at once. It is no good waiting for disappointing results and then telling everyone that you felt ghastly at the time but said nothing to anyone. Exam boards can give you special consideration if the appropriate forms are sent to them by the school, along with supporting evidence.

Your extenuating circumstances must be convincing. A 'slight sniffle' won't do! If you really are sufficiently ill to be unable to prepare for the exams or to perform effectively during them, you must consult your GP and obtain a letter describing your condition.

The other main cause of under-performance is distressing events at home. If a member of your immediate family is very seriously ill, you should explain this to your headteacher and persuade him or her to write to the examiners and medical schools.

With luck, the exam board will give you the benefit of the doubt if your marks fall on a grade border. Equally, you can hope that the medical school will allow you to slip one grade below the conditional offer. If things work out badly, then the fact that you declared extenuating circumstances should ensure that you are treated sympathetically when you reapply through UCAS. This point is covered in more detail in 'What to do when you get your results' (page 48).

WHAT TO DO WHEN YOU GET YOUR RESULTS

The A-level results will arrive at your school on the third Thursday in August. The medical schools will have received them a few days earlier. You must make sure that you are at home on the day the results are published. Don't wait for the school to post the results slip to you. Get the staff to tell you the news as soon as possible. If you need to act to secure a place, you may have to act quickly.

The medical school admissions departments are well organised and efficient, but they are staffed by human beings. If there were extenuating circumstances that could have affected your exam performance and which were brought to their notice in June, it is a good idea to ask them to review the relevant letters shortly before the exam results are published.

If you previously received a conditional offer and your grades equal or exceed that offer, congratulations! You can relax and wait for your chosen medical school to send you joining instructions. One word of warning: you cannot assume that grades of AAC satisfy an ABB offer. This is especially true if the C grade is in chemistry. Read on.

The paragraphs that follow take you through the steps you should follow if you need to use the Clearing system because you have good grades but no offer. They also explain what to do if your grades are disappointing.

WHAT TO DO IF YOU HAVE GOOD GRADES BUT NO OFFER

Every year, UCAS statistics reveal that between 400 and 500 people get into medical school through Clearing. However, that does not mean that all of these were students who were not holding offers but who nevertheless gained places – many of these were students who narrowly missed their offers, but were given places based on their strong performance at interview or because of extenuating circumstances. Table 2 (page 83) shows that very few schools keep places open and, of those that do, most will choose to allow applicants who hold a conditional offer to slip a grade rather than dust off a reserve list of those they interviewed but didn't make an offer to. Still less are they likely to consider applicants who appear out of the blue – however high their grades. That said, it is likely that every summer a few medical schools will have enough unfilled places to consider a Clearing-style application.

If you hold three A grades but were rejected when you applied through UCAS you need to let the medical schools know that you are out there. The best way to do this is by fax. Fax and phone numbers are listed in the UCAS Directory. If you live nearby, you can always deliver a letter in person, talk to the office staff and hope that your application will stand out from the rest.

Set out opposite is a sample letter/fax. Don't copy it word for word!

Don't forget that your UCAS referee may be able to help you. Try to persuade him or her to ring the admissions officers on your behalf – he or she will find it easier to get through than you will. If your headteacher is unable/unwilling to ring, then he or she should, at least, fax a note in support of your application. It is best if both faxes arrive at the medical school at the same time.

If you are applying to a medical school that did not receive your UCAS form, ask your head to fax or send a copy of the form. In general, it is best to persuade the medical school to invite you to arrange for the UCAS form to be sent.

If, despite your most strenuous efforts, you are unsuccessful, you need to consider applying again (see below). The other alternative is to use the Clearing system to obtain a place on a degree course related to medicine and hope to be accepted on the medical course after you graduate. This option is described on page 57.

```
                                                    Your name
                                                     Address
                                              Telephone number

Date

The Admissions Officer (by name if possible)
St James's Hospital Medical School
Address

Dear (name)              UCAS No. 1234567

I have just received my A-level results which were:

        Biology A, Chemistry A, English A

I also have a B Grade in AS Philosophy

You may remember that I applied to St James's but was rejected after
interview/was rejected without an interview. I am still very keen to study
medicine at St James's and hope that you will consider me for any places
which may now be available.

My headteacher supports my application and is faxing you a note to this
effect. Should you wish to contact him, the details are: Mr W F Smith,
Tel: 0123 456 7891, Fax: 0123 456 7892.

I can be contacted at the above address and could attend an interview at
short notice.

Yours sincerely

[Your signature]

Your name
```

WHAT TO DO IF YOU HOLD AN OFFER BUT YOUR GRADES ARE DISAPPOINTING

The options

If you have only narrowly missed the required grades (this includes the
AAC grade case described above), it is important that you and your

referee fax the medical school to put your case before you are rejected. Another sample letter follows below.

Your name
Address
Telephone number

Date

The Admissions Officer (by name if possible)
St James's Hospital Medical School
Address

Dear (name)   **UCAS No. 1234567**

I have just received my A-level results which were:

Chemistry A, Biology A, English C

I also have a B Grade in AS Photography

I hold a conditional offer from St James's of ABB and I realise that my grades fall below that offer. Nevertheless I am still determined to study medicine and I hope you will be able to find a place for me this year.

May I remind you that at the time of the exams I was recovering from glandular fever. A medical certificate to this effect was sent to you in June by my headteacher.

My headteacher supports my application and is faxing you a note to this effect. Should you wish to contact him, the details are: Mr W F Smith, Tel: 0123 456 7891, Fax: 0123 456 7892.

I can be contacted at the above address and could attend an interview at short notice.

Yours sincerely

[Your signature]

Your name

If this is unsuccessful, you need to consider retaking your A-levels and applying again (page 52). The other alternative is to use the Clearing system to obtain a place on a degree course related to medicine and hope to apply to the medical course after you graduate. This option is described on page 57.

Retaking your A-level(s)

The grade requirements for retake candidates are normally higher than for first timers (usually AAA). You should retake any subject where your first result was below B and you should aim for an A grade in any subject you do retake. It is often necessary to retake a B grade, especially in chemistry – take advice from the college that is preparing you for the retake.

Most AS and A2 units or modules can be taken in January sittings, and some boards offer other sittings. This means that a January retake is often technically possible, although you should check carefully before taking up this option, since there may be complications because of the number of times units/modules have been already taken, and because of coursework.

The timescale for your retake will depend on:

- the grades you obtained first time
- the syllabuses you studied.

If you simply need to improve one subject by one or two grades and can retake the exam on the same syllabus in January, then the short retake course is the logical option.

If, on the other hand, your grades were DDE and you took your exams through a board which has no midyear retakes for the units that you require, you probably need to spend another year on your retakes. You would find it almost impossible to master syllabus changes in three subjects and achieve an increase of nine or ten grades within the 17 weeks that are available for teaching between September and January.

Independent sixth-form colleges provide specialist advice and teaching for students considering A-level retakes. Interviews to discuss this are free and carry no obligation to enrol on a course, so it is worth taking the time to talk to their staff before you embark on A-level retakes.

Reapplying to medical school

Many medical schools discourage retake candidates (see Table 1, page 81) so the whole business of applying again needs careful thought, hard work and a bit of luck.

The choice of medical schools for your UCAS form is narrower than it was the first time round. Don't apply to the medical schools that discourage retakers unless there really are special, extenuating circumstances to explain your disappointing grades. Among the excuses that will not wash are:

'I wasn't feeling too good on the day of the practical exam, knocked over my Bunsen and torched the answer book.'

'My dog had been ill for a week before my exams and only recovered after the last paper (and I've got a vet's certificate to prove it).'

'I'd spent the month before the exams condensing my notes onto small cards so that I could revise effectively. Two days before the exams our house was broken into and the burglar trod on my notes as he climbed through the window. The police took them away for forensic examination and didn't give them back until after the last paper (and I've got a note from the CID to prove it).'

Some reasons are acceptable to even the most fanatical opponents of retake candidates:

■ your own illness
■ the death or serious illness of a very close relative.

Consider, in addition, your age when you took the exams. Most medical schools will accept that a candidate who was well under the age of 18 on the date of sitting A-levels may deserve another attempt without being branded as a 'retaker'.

These are just guidelines and the only safe method of finding out if a medical school will accept you is to write and ask them. A typical letter is set out on the following page. Don't follow it slavishly and do take the time to write to several medical schools before you make your final choice.

Your name
Address
Telephone number

Date

The Admissions Officer (by name if possible)
St James's Hospital Medical School
Address

Dear Sir/Madam   **Last Year's UCAS No. 1234567**

I am writing to ask your advice because I am about to complete my UCAS form and would very much like to apply to St James's.

You may remember that I applied to you last year and received an offer of AAB/was rejected after interview/was rejected without an interview.

I have just received my A-level results which were:

> Biology C, Chemistry D, English E

I also have a B Grade in AS Psychology

I was aged 17 years and six months at the time of taking these exams.

I plan to retake Chemistry in January after a 17-week course and English over a year. If necessary, I will retake Biology in the period from January to June. I am confident that I can push these subjects up to A grades overall.

What worries me is that I have heard that some medical schools do not consider retake candidates even when the exams were taken under the age of 18 and relatively high grades were obtained. I am very keen not to waste a slot on my UCAS form (or your time) by applying to schools that will reject me purely because I am retaking.

I am very keen to come to St James's and would be extremely grateful for any advice that you can give me.

Yours faithfully

[Your signature]

Your name

Notice that the format of your letter should be:

- opening paragraph
- your exam results – set out clearly and with no omissions
- any extenuating circumstances – a brief statement
- your retake plan – including the timescale
- a request for help and advice
- closing paragraph.

Make sure that your letter is brief, clear and well presented. You can type or word-process it, if you wish, but you should write 'Dear Sir/Madam' and 'Yours faithfully' by hand. If you have had any previous contact with the admissions staff you will be able to write 'Dear Dr Smith' and 'Yours sincerely'. Even if you go to this trouble the pressure on medical schools in the autumn is such that you may receive no more than a photocopied standard reply to the effect that, if you apply, your application will be considered.

Apart from the care needed in making the choice of medical school, the rest of the application procedure is as described in the first part of this guide.

NON-STANDARD APPLICATIONS

So far, this guide has been concerned with the 'standard' applicant: the UK resident who is studying at least two science subjects at A-level and who is applying from school or who is retaking immediately after disappointing A-levels. Medical schools accept a small number of applicants who do not have this 'standard' background. The main non-standard categories are as follows.

THOSE WHO HAVE NOT STUDIED SCIENCE A-LEVELS

If you decide that you would like to study medicine after having already started on a combination of A-levels that does not fit the subject requirements for entry to medical school, you can apply for the 'premedical course'. This is offered at eight university faculties of medicine.

The course covers elements of chemistry, biology and physics and lasts one academic year. It leads to the first MB qualification for which science A-levels provide exemption.

If your pre-med application is rejected, you will have to spend a further two years taking science A-levels at a sixth-form college. Independent sixth-form colleges offer one-year A-level courses and certain subjects can be covered from scratch in a single year. However, only very able students can cover A-level chemistry and biology in a single year with good results. You should discuss your particular circumstances with the staff of a number of colleges in order to select the course that will prepare you to achieve the A-level subjects you need at the grades you require.

OVERSEAS STUDENTS

Most medical schools are limited by government quota to accepting only 7.5 per cent of overseas students each year. In the academic year 2002/2003 the tuition fees charged to these students were typically between £10,000 and £12,000 per year for the pre-clinical and between £19,000 and £20,000 per year for the clinical courses.

The competition for the few places available to overseas students is fierce and you would be wise to discuss your application informally with the medical school before submitting your UCAS form. Many medical schools give preference to students who do not have adequate provision for training in their own countries. You should contact the medical schools individually for advice.

Information about qualifications can be obtained from British Council offices, or British Embassies.

MATURE STUDENTS AND GRADUATES

Each year a small percentage of the entrants to medicine are aged 22–30 (see Table 2, page 83). In exceptional circumstances, candidates who are over 30 may be considered. In general, there are two types of mature applicant:

- those who have always wanted to study medicine but who failed to get into medical school when they applied from school in the normal way
- those who came to the idea later on in life, often having embarked on a totally different career.

The first type of mature applicant has usually followed a degree course in a subject related to medicine, obtained a good grade (minimum 2.1) and hopes to gain some exemption from part of the pre-clinical course. These students have an uphill path into medicine because their early failure tends to prejudice the selectors. Nevertheless, they do not have the problem of taking science A-levels at a late stage in their education. If you want to follow this option you should apply through Clearing for one of the medically related degrees, such as:

- Anatomy
- Biomedical Sciences

- Biochemistry
- Human Biology
- Medical Science
- Pharmacology
- Physiology.

The second category of mature student is often of more interest to the medical school selectors and interviewers. Applications from people aged under 30 who have achieved success in other careers and who can bring a breadth of experience to the medical school and to the profession are welcomed.

The main difficulty facing those who come late to the idea of studying medicine is that they rarely have a scientific background. They face the daunting task of studying science A-levels and need very careful counselling before they embark on what will, inevitably, be quite a tough programme. Independent sixth-form colleges provide this counselling as part of their normal interview procedure.

GRADUATE COURSES

The biggest change in medical school entry in recent years has been the development of graduate entry schemes. The first medical schools to introduce an accelerated course specifically for graduates were St George's Hospital Medical School and Leicester/Warwick. The St George's course, in particular, has gained a good deal of publicity through a 'fly on the wall' documentary, *Help! I'm a Doctor*, which followed four graduates as they embarked upon their medical training. A number of medical schools now operate graduate schemes, including Birmingham, Cambridge, Leicester/Warwick, Liverpool, Newcastle, Nottingham, Oxford, and Queen Mary and Westfield. Entry for some of these courses is through a combination of examination (the GAMSAT exam) and interview. By the UCAS deadline of 15 October, nearly 3000 of the 14,000 applicants had applied for four-year graduate entry courses.

ACCESS COURSES

Another recent development has been the growth of courses that allow direct access to medical school for mature students or students who have not followed the traditional academic paths to medical school entry. Two notable schemes are those set up by the College of West Anglia in King's Lynn, and by King's College. The College of West Anglia course has an impressive track record in placing mature students at medical schools throughout the country. The success rate of the one-year course is extremely high (over 90 per cent), and assessment is through coursework as well as by examination. The course is recognised by more than half of the UK medical schools. Contact details can be found at the end of this book. The King's College course is a six-year programme that has been designed to help students living in five inner London boroughs. Students are selected on the basis of potential rather than actual performance at A-level. Details can be found at the end of the book.

Mature students are wise to seek an informal chat with the medical school admissions staff before submitting their UCAS forms.

STUDYING OUTSIDE THE UK

If you are unsuccessful in gaining a place at one of the UK medical schools, and do not want to follow the graduate-entry path, you might want to look at other options. There are medical schools throughout the world that will accept A-level students, but the important issue is whether or not you would be able, should you wish to do so, to practise in the UK upon qualification. Popular courses for UK students are:

- Royal College of Surgeons in Dublin. Students from countries within the European Union who qualify gain limited registration from the GMC.
- St George's University School of Medicine in Grenada (West Indies). Students who wish to practise in the UK can spend part of the clinical stage of the course in a range of hospitals in the UK including GKT in London. To practise in the UK, students sit the UEB, an examination equivalent to the qualification examination set by UK medical schools. Clinical experience can also be gained in hospitals in the US, allowing students to practise there as well. A high proportion of the medical school teachers have worked in UK universities and medical schools.
- Medical courses taught in English, at Charles University in Prague and at other universities in the Czech Republic.

Details of these medical schools can be found in the 'Useful addresses' section at the end of the book.

CURRENT ISSUES

GOVERNMENT REFORMS OF THE NHS

A little history to set the scene

The National Health Service was set up in 1948 to provide healthcare free of charge at the point of delivery. This is not to say that, if you fell ill in 1947, you necessarily had to pay for your treatment. Accident and emergency services had been developed and had coped well with the demands of a population under bombardment during the world war. Some hospitals were ancient and wealthy charitable institutions owning valuable assets such as property in London. These hospitals charged patients who could afford to pay and treated others without charge. Doctors often worked on the same basis. Other hospitals were owned and funded by local authorities. The system was supported by low-cost insurance schemes which were often fully or partially funded by employers.

The problem perceived by the architects of the NHS was that poorer members of society were reluctant to seek diagnosis and treatment. By funding the system out of a national insurance scheme to which every employer and employee would contribute, the government conferred on all citizens (whether employed or not) the right to free healthcare without stigma. However, even at the beginning there were two drawbacks:

- The introduction of the NHS was not universally popular among the medical profession.
- While it conferred rights, the NHS imposed no duties on the users of the system. Consequently some patients made (and continue to make) unreasonable demands, for example, by requesting home visits at night for non-emergency conditions.

The service has undergone a number of reforms since 1948, but by far the most fundamental was introduced by the Conservative government in

1990. It is important to understand what these reforms were, why they were thought to be necessary and what the outcome has been.

By the late 1980s it was clear to the government that the NHS could not function in the future without a substantial increase in funding. The fundamental reason for this was the expected reduction in the supply of money from taxpayers linked to an anticipated increase in demand for healthcare. Let's see why this was so.

Increased demand
By 1990:

- The NHS had become a victim of its own success; when the service saved the life of a patient who would normally have died, that person survived to have another illness, to receive more treatment and incur more expense for the NHS.
- The number of life-prolonging procedures/treatments/drugs had increased as a result of developments in medical science.
- The cost of these sophisticated procedures/treatments/drugs was high and increasing at a rate faster than inflation.
- The cost of staff had increased because, while rates of pay had increased, the hours worked for that pay had fallen. Simultaneously, the cost of training staff in the new procedures and equipment was high.
- Patient expectations had risen. Knowledge of the new procedures/treatment/drugs meant that patients demanded access to them without delay.

A solution to the problem

The government believed that there were inefficiencies in the NHS which, if removed, would counter the pressure on funds and they resolved to use market forces to overcome these inefficiencies.

What are market forces? If in 1985 (before the fall of Communism) you had travelled to Moscow and tried to buy an orange in a government food store, you would have faced a long queue. When you reached the end of the queue you would have found that the oranges were of poor quality and very expensive. Back in London, you would have found it easy to buy oranges – they were plentiful, of good quality and cheap. The reason for the difference was market forces: in the Soviet Union there was no free market – the state decided how many oranges were to be grown, where they were to be sold and at what price. In a free market, on the other hand, individual traders compete with each other to sell more oranges and this competition keeps quality up and costs down, according to public demand.

Applying the market to the NHS

For a market to work you need providers (of goods and services) and purchasers. The purchasers need the freedom to choose between several providers and extensive information about the price and quality of the goods or services offered by each provider.

Logically, therefore, the government should have given us back our taxes and left us free to shop around for the best deals. We could have chosen the hospital that offered us the cheapest hip replacement operation and kept the change. Of course that isn't what they did, governments give back taxes as willingly as water flows uphill and, anyway, there is a significant section of the population that pays no tax. Instead, they asked the District Health Authorities and the General Practitioners (GPs) to act as purchasers on our behalf and, by doing so, they began to water down the principle of the market and, arguably, its benefits.

The scheme was designed to work as follows.

Hospital trusts
Before the reforms hospitals were operated and funded by District Health Authorities (DHAs). The government wanted the DHAs, and later the GPs, to become 'purchasers' and the hospitals to become 'providers' in the new health marketplace. Hospitals (or groups of hospitals) were told to form themselves into NHS Trusts which would act as independent businesses but with a number of crucial and (market diluting) differences. They were to calculate the cost of all the treatment they offered and to price it at cost to the GP purchasers. In addition, and on the assumption that there were inefficiencies within the system that needed to be weeded out, they were told to reduce this cost by 3 per cent annually.

GP fundholders

GPs were encouraged to become 'fundholders'. Historically, GPs have received money according to a formula based largely on the number and age of the patients registered with them. In addition, these fundholders were now to receive annually a sum of money (the fund) based on the cost of hospital treatment and prescribed drugs received by their patients. They were to be empowered to buy hospital treatment for their patients at the best price they could find. If they could do this at a total cost lower than the fund, they could invest the surplus in their 'practice' for the benefit of their patients. The fundholding scheme was not designed to cover the cost of acute emergency work.

Rational prescribing of drugs by their generic names

In 1989 drugs cost £1.9 billion, more than the cost of the GPs themselves. In order to achieve savings, GPs were encouraged to be more aware of the cost of the drugs they were prescribing and to bear in mind the possibility that a 'generic' version of the drug might do the same job at a cheaper price. For example, Glaxo-Wellcome's best-selling drug 'Zantac' is now no longer protected by patents and other manufacturers are free to produce a drug with the same active ingredient which is known by the generic name of 'Ranitidine'.

What happened in practice

The cost of treatment

Even after over ten years of the internal market, there are still dramatic differences in the treatments available on a regional basis. There are also wide variations in the cost of operations between hospitals. The Department of Health figures released in January 2000 highlighted the range of costs for the 20 million hospital treatments carried out in 1998/99. For instance, the average cost of an appendix operation was £1127, but the cost varied from £50 in one hospital to £7460 in another.

The hospitals

The effect of the reforms was dramatic and largely unpopular. The most unpopular was the assertion that old hospitals in areas of low population density were not economically viable and should be closed. St Bartholomew's Hospital in the City of London was an example.

Suddenly there were winners and losers in a world which had considered itself removed from the pressures of commercial life.

As doctors faced up to the possibility that ancient institutions could be closed down and the centres of medical expertise built up over generations dispersed, they were less than thrilled to observe the huge influx of cost accountants and client service officers – the bureaucracy that was necessary to ensure that the new hospital trusts could measure the costs they were charging out to GP fundholders. Putting this into perspective, by 1994:

- the number of managers in the health service had increased from 4610 to 16,690
- the number of clerical and administrative staff had gone from 18,000 to 134,990
- the overall bill for senior managers had risen from £30m to £383m.

It should be recognised that some of these 'managers' were people already working in the NHS who had been reclassified: ward sisters had become ward managers. Furthermore, some of the desired efficiencies have been achieved even if, as some doctors now argue, staffing levels have fallen and bed occupancy rates risen to the point where patients are being put at risk.

The GPs
By the middle of 1997, 15,000 GP practices (one in two) were fundholding, but the Audit Commission reported that the benefits to patients had been marginal – hospital waiting lists for the patients of fundholders and non-fundholders were roughly the same.

The cost of the fundholder scheme (about £250m) has been criticised, as has the amount of money spent on processing invoices. A health authority in the south processed 60,000 invoices per year, representing 8 per cent of its healthcare budget, and an inner city trust dealing with over 900 funds had to send out over 40,000 invoices per year.

Care in the community

Another controversial aspect of the NHS reforms, and one that has had a great impact on GP workload, has been the decision to transfer as many patients as possible from secondary (hospital) care to primary (community) care. In practice, this has led to the decision to close down many of the old mental and other long-stay hospitals and release the patients to be 'cared for in the community'. The argument is that it is inhuman to lock up patients in 'Victorian' institutions when they could enjoy quasi-normal lives.

The system has worked well in some cases but the release of schizophrenics who, free of close supervision, have failed to take the drugs that control their dangerous condition is a cause of concern. It has been estimated that, on average, two people are murdered every month by mentally ill people who have been released into the community. It is argued that community care can only function properly if it is properly funded and that proper funding would be more expensive than building new secure hospitals for the mentally ill. The Mental Health Foundation estimates that an extra £540m is needed annually to provide adequate care for the 300,000 severely mentally ill.

The drugs bill

One of the great successes of the reforms has been savings in the GP drugs bill. Every GP now receives a quarterly statement from the 'Prescription Pricing Authority' which lists the prescribing costs in the practice and compares them with the costs in the local area and in the country as a whole. It analyses spending by therapeutic group (eg the cardiovascular system) and by individual drug. Where a generic equivalent is available that fact is indicated. At the same time it has 'blacklisted' drugs that are considered ineffective. A typical London GP practice saved £100,000 annually as a result of prescribing decisions based on this information.

Inevitably, even this story has its flip side. Three concerns are:

- Doctors worry that generic equivalents produced cheaply outside the UK do not conform to our expectations of purity.
- These savings hit the profits of the international pharmaceutical companies which may then find it harder to fund research into new drugs and may be less inclined to site their research and production facilities in the UK.
- The government has increased prescription charges (the amount you pay the pharmacist for the drug prescribed by your GP) to the point

where it is often cheaper to buy it yourself. Not surprisingly, the government has also worked to move some drugs off the list of drugs that can only be issued on prescription and make them available 'over the counter'.

The White Paper – December 1997

The New NHS: Modern, Dependable – the Government White Paper of 1997 – made a number of suggestions.

- The replacement of the Internal Market with 'Integrated Care'. This involved the formation of 500 Primary Care Groups typically covering 100,000 patients – bringing together family doctors and community nurses – replacing GP fundholding, which ceased to exist in 1999.
- NHSnet. Every GP surgery and hospital will be connected via the Internet. It will mean less waiting for prescriptions, quicker appointments, and less delay in getting results of tests.
- New services for patients. Everyone with suspected cancer will be guaranteed an appointment with a specialist within two weeks.
- NHS Direct. A 24-hour nurse-led telephone advice and information service.
- Savings. £1 billion savings from cutting paperwork, which will be ploughed back into patient care.

Rationing and NICE

'Rationing' of healthcare causes particular concern amongst the population. The issue hit the headlines in January 1999 when Frank Dobson (who was Health Secretary at the time) announced that, because of lack of funds, the use of Viagra (an anti-impotence drug) would be rationed: the NHS would only provide Viagra for cases of impotence arising from a small number of named causes. To take an example, a man whose impotence was caused by diabetes could be provided with Viagra on the NHS, whereas if the cause had been kidney failure, he would have to pay for the drug privately.

The publicity surrounding Viagra alerted people to other issues, in particular:

- *Rationing by age*

  The charity Age Concern commissioned a Gallup poll which, they claim, revealed that older people were being denied healthcare and being poorly treated in both primary and secondary care. The BMA responded by arguing that people of different ages require different patterns of treatment or referral. They cited the example of the progression of cancer, which is more rapid in younger people and often needs more aggressive radiotherapy, chemotherapy or surgery.

- *Postcode prescribing*

  Until the formation of NICE (see below) in 1999, health authorities received little guidance in what drugs and treatments to prescribe. Some well-publicised cases revealed large differences in the range of drugs and treatments available between regions (hence the term 'postcode rationing'). Beta interferon, a drug that extended the remission from MS in some patients, was prescribed by some health authorities but not by others, and the press highlighted cases where patients were forced to pay thousands of pounds a year to buy the drug privately, when others at an identical stage of MS but who lived a few miles away, received the drug on the NHS.

NICE

The National Institute for Clinical Excellence (NICE) was set up as a Special Health Authority in April 1999. Its role is to provide the NHS with guidance on individual health technologies (for instance, drugs) and treatments. In the words of the Chairman of NICE, Professor Sir Michael Rawlins, *'NICE is about taking a look at what's available, identifying what works and helping the NHS to get more of what works into practice'*. The government has acknowledged that there are variations in the quality of care available to different patients in different parts of the country, and it hopes that the guidance that NICE can provide will reduce these differences. In a speech explaining the role of NICE, the Chairman said that it has been estimated that, on average, health professionals should be reading 19 medical and scientific articles each day if they are to keep up to date – in future, they can read the NICE bulletins instead. It is unlikely, however, that NICE will end the controversies surrounding new treatments, since it will not only be making recommendations based on clinical effectiveness, but also on cost effectiveness – something that is very difficult to judge. A good example of a situation where a drug can be clinically effective but not cost effective is the case of the first drug that NICE reviewed, a new treatment for influenza, called zanamivir (Relenza). Despite a hefty publicity campaign when it was introduced, NICE advised doctors and health authorities not to prescribe the drug. NICE argued that although the clinical trials showed that, if taken within 48 hours of the onset of symptoms, the duration of 'flu is reduced by 24 hours, there was no evidence that it would save the lives of the 3000–4000 deaths a year which result from complications from 'flu.

In addition to Relenza, NICE has investigated the effectiveness of many treatments including:

- Hip replacement joints
- Therapy for depression
- Crohn's Disease
- Coronary artery stents
- Drugs for Hepatitis C
- Surgery for corectal cancer
- Drugs (Taxanes) for breast cancer
- Drugs (Temozolomide) for brain cancer
- Inhaler systems for children with asthma.

Full details of the results of these, and other investigations, can be found on the NICE website (www.nice.org.uk).

SARS

The biggest medical story in recent months has been the arrival of a previously unknown respiratory illness called Severe Acute Respiratory Syndrome (SARS). SARS has affected people in Asia, North America and Europe, with China reporting the most cases. SARS begins with a fever and other symptoms may include headache, an overall feeling of discomfort, and body aches. Some people also experience mild respiratory symptoms. After 2 to 7 days, SARS patients may develop a dry cough and have trouble breathing.

SARS appears to spread by close person-to-person contact. Most cases have involved people who cared for or lived with someone with SARS, or had direct contact with infectious material (for example, respiratory secretions) from a person who has SARS. The SARS virus is a previously unrecognised coronavirus.

By the middle of May 2003, the World Health Organisation reported about 7500 cases of SARS worldwide, with 600 deaths attributed to the illness. These figures probably underestimate the effect of SARS since there is some evidence that a number of countries have tried to play down the scale of the problem.

Research published in *The Lancet* medical journal in May 2003 suggested that SARS is more deadly than many other respiratory diseases, particularly for older patients. *The Lancet* reported that SARS is killing one in five of patients with the virus in hard-hit Hong Kong, including 55 per cent of infected patients aged over 60. In younger patients, the death rate could be as low as 6.8 per cent, the study found.

An update on SARS can be found on the *Getting into Medical School* website.

MAD COWS, ETC

The continuing publicity given to the problems associated with mad cow disease and the interesting nature of the infectious agent make it a common topic for interview questions.

1. What is 'mad cow disease'?
The scientific name is bovine spongiform encephalopathy (BSE). The disease converts the brain of the affected animal into a spongy form which prevents normal functioning.

2. Where did it come from?
An equivalent disease has existed for a long time in sheep where it is called scrapie. It is thought, but not proved, that cows became affected because they were fed with sheep products which had not been properly sterilised.

3. What is the human form called?
A human spongiform encephalopathy was identified by two German doctors, Creutzfeldt and Jakob, after whom it is named. They identified CJD in the 1920s. The classic form attacks the elderly and is rare: it affects only one person in a million. A new form of CJD has recently

been reported in the UK. This new form affects young healthy adults and has been linked with BSE. Officially, the new form had claimed 35 lives up to the beginning of 1999.

4. What is thought to be the infectious agent?

Whereas disease is normally transmitted by bacteria or viruses, the spongiform encephalopathies are thought to be transmitted by prions: misshapen proteins. Because prions are distortions of the body's own protein they do not trigger the immune system. Worryingly, they seem to be unaffected by either heat or radiation.

5. Can CJD be treated ?

At present there is no treatment. All who develop CJD die of the disease.

6. Can humans become infected with CJD as a result of eating sheep products?

Interestingly, there is no suggestion that humans have ever become infected as a result of eating sheep products.

7. Can humans become infected with CJD as a result of eating beef products?

A good question! One of the ironies of the BSE/CJD crisis is that there is no causal evidence to link the onset of CJD with eating beef. The circumstantial evidence is:

- The new form of CJD coincided with an epidemic of BSE in Britain.
- Scientists believe that BSE originated in scrapie and that scrapie was transmitted when cows were fed with infected sheep products.
- There is a CJD-like disease called Kuru in Papua New Guinea. It is believed that this disease is spread when the inhabitants eat the brains of their dead relatives – a traditional custom.
- Injecting material from cows suffering with BSE into the brains of macaque monkeys produces patterns of brain damage similar to those seen in patients suffering from the new variant of CJD.

8. What happens next?

The steps taken to control BSE reduced the incidence of the disease from more than 35,000 cases in 1992 to about 1300 cases in 2000. It is hoped that the disease will be almost eliminated within a few years. If BSE-affected beef and other products are removed from the human food chain, and so long as there is no general fashion for cannibalism, the new prions should die with their hosts. The danger is that new CJD is in the human population. The prions have no genes but might find some way to adapt to their new surroundings which would permit them a new method of transmission. There is a suspicion that CJD could be passed on through blood transfusions, and for this reason, the USA has banned the use of blood donated by people who spent 'a significant' time in the UK in the late 1980s and early 1990s. In 1997, the government set up a public inquiry, chaired by Lord Philips. The findings were released in October 2000. Details can be found on the inquiry website (www.bseinquiry.gov.uk).

The BSE problem raised a number of issues concerning farming and food safety. In retrospect, the decision to allow the remains of diseased animals to be incorporated into animal feed seems to be misguided, at the very least. The problem with BSE is that the infecting agent, the prion (a previously unknown pathogen composed of proteins) was able to survive the treatments used to destroy bacteria and viruses. If any good has come out of the problem, it is that we are now much more aware of food safety. In April 2000, the government established the Food Standards Agency, created to 'protect public health from risks which may arise in connection with the consumption of food, and otherwise to protect the interests of consumers in relation to food'. Although it has been established by the government, it has the independence to publish any advice that it gives the government, avoiding the accusations of cover-ups and secrecy levelled at the government over the BSE affair.

GENES – MEDICAL AND ETHICAL ASPECTS

Gene therapy and the Human Genome Project

Many illnesses are thought to be caused by defective genes: examples are cancer, cystic fibrosis and Alzheimer's disease. The defects may be hereditary or triggered by external factors such as ionising or solar radiation. The much-hyped dream of medical researchers, especially in the USA, is that the affected chromosomes could be repaired, allowing the body to heal itself.

71

To make this dream come true, the therapist needs to know which gene is causing the problem and how to replace it with a healthy one. Great progress has been made in solving the first part of the puzzle thanks to a gigantic international research project known as the 'Human Genome Project' which has, as its aim, the identification of every human gene and an understanding of what effect it has. The full sequence was published in early 2000. Many links have been made between diseases and specific genes but the techniques for replacing the defective genes have yet to prove themselves.

Two methods have been proposed:

- The healthy gene is incorporated in a retro-virus which, by its nature, splices its genetic material into the chromosomes of the host cell. The virus must first be treated in order to prevent it causing problems of its own. This 'denaturing' reduces the positive effects and, to date, the trials have been unconvincing.
- The healthy gene is incorporated in a fatty droplet which is sprayed into the nose in order to reach cells in the lining of the nose, air passages and lungs, or injected into the blood. It was hoped that this method would be effective against the single defective gene that causes cystic fibrosis but, again, the trials have yet to prove successful.

To make matters worse, it turns out that many of the illnesses which are genetic in origin are caused by defects in a wide number of genes so that the hoped-for magic bullet needs to be replaced by a magic cluster bomb and that sounds suspiciously like the approach used by conventional pharmaceuticals. Since 1990, when gene therapy for humans began, about 300 clinical trials (involving diseases ranging from cystic fibrosis and heart disease to brain tumours) have been carried out, with very limited success.

Genetic engineering

Genetic engineering is the name given to the manipulation of genes. There is a subtle difference between genetic engineering and gene therapy. Specifically, genetic engineering implies modification of the genes involved in reproduction. These modifications will then be carried over into future generations.

One of the reasons for considering these ideas is to try to produce enhanced performance in animals and plants. The possibility of applying genetic engineering to humans poses major ethical problems and, at present, experiments involving reproductive cells are prohibited. Nevertheless, one form of genetic engineering known as genetic screening is allowed. In this technique, an egg is fertilised in a test tube. When the embryo is two days old, one cell is removed and the chromosomes are tested to establish the sex and presence of gene defects. In the light of the tests, the parents decide whether or not to implant the embryo into the mother's womb.

Taken to its logical conclusion, this is the recipe for creating a breed of supermen. The superman concept may be morally acceptable when applied to race horses, but should it be applied to merchant bankers? How would we feel if a small undemocratic state decided to apply this strategy to its entire population in order to obtain an economic advantage? Could we afford to ignore this challenge?

The fundamental argument against any policy that reduces variation in the human gene pool is that it is intrinsically dangerous because, in principle, it restricts the species' ability to adapt to new environmental challenges. Inability to adapt to an extreme challenge could lead to extinction of our species.

Human Cloning

In December 2002, a cult-linked company called Clonaid announced that the first human cloned baby had been born, and that three more were due in January. Whilst there is no evidence that this actually occurred, it did bring the issue of human cloning back into the news (and, incidentally, back on to the agenda for medical school interview questions).

Reasons why people may want human cloning:

- Infertility
- 'Recover' a child who has died
- Eugenics – to improve the human race
- Spare parts
- Research purposes.

Reasons why people are against human cloning:

- Health risks from mutation of genes
- Risks of abuse of the technology
- Ethical/religious reasons
- Emotional risks for cloned child.

Dolly the sheep

Dolly, born at the Roslin Institute in Edinburgh, hit the headlines in February 1997 because she was the first mammal to be cloned from an adult cell. The importance of the birth is not the fact that a sheep had been cloned, as this had been done before using embryo cells, but that nobody had successfully taken adult cells – in this case from the udder of a six-year-old ewe – and cloned them.

Embryo cells have the potential to become complete embryos, but adult cells are differentiated – for instance, cells in the liver do the job of the liver – and so cloning is much more difficult. The process begins by starving cells of nutrients for a few days until they stop growing and dividing. The nucleus of one of these quiescent cells is then injected into a cell which had previously had its nucleus removed. A small electric current is used to kick the cell back into activity, and it is then put into the womb of a female sheep to grow. The egg now contains a full set of genes, as if it had been fertilised by a spermatozoa. It took 277 attempts to produce the first successful clone.

The difference between cloning and IVF treatment is that, in the latter, eggs are fertilised in a test tube (hence the so-called 'test-tube babies') using sperm from a male, and then placed in the uterus; whereas cloning involves the removal of the egg nucleus which is then replaced by the nucleus of the cell which is to be cloned. A cloned animal has only one parent.

Cloning could be an important source of genetically identical copies of organs, skin and blood cells for surgical use. The biotechnology company, PPL Therapeutics, that worked with the Roslin scientists hopes to use the cloning technique to produce sheep capable of generating the blood-clotting protein Factor IX in their milk. PPL estimates that 50 sheep would be enough to produce the £100m annual world demand for Factor IX. In January 2002 it was discovered that Dolly had arthritis. It is unusual for sheep under six years old to get arthritis in the rear legs, and this has raised fears that premature ageing could be the result of cloning. There is also chromosome evidence that Dolly aged faster than non-cloned sheep. If organs from cloned animals are one day going to be used for human transplants, will they age prematurely in the human's body?

On Friday 14 February 2003, Dolly was put down at the relatively young age of six years old, because the scientists decided that she would not recover from a progressive lung disease. Dr Harry Griffin, the acting Director at Roslin, said: 'Sheep can live to 11 or 12 years of age, and lung diseases are common in older sheep, particularly those housed indoors. There is no evidence that cloning was a factor in Dolly contracting the disease.'

The post-mortem did not uncover any other abnormalities.

WORLD HEALTH: RICH VS POOR

In the industrialised world, infectious diseases are well under control. The main threats to health are circulatory diseases (such as heart disease and stroke), cancer, respiratory ailments and musculoskeletal conditions (rheumatic diseases and osteoporosis). All of these are diseases which tend to affect older people and, as life expectancy is increasing, they will become more prevalent in the future. Many are nutrition-related, where an unhealthy diet rich in saturated fats and processed foods leads to poor health.

In poorer countries, infectious diseases such as malaria, cholera, tuberculosis, hepatitis and HIV/AIDS are much more common. Malaria affects up to 500 million people a year and kills over a million; and 1.5 million die from tuberculosis. The UN estimated that in 2002, there were 42 million people infected with HIV/AIDS and over 3 million people died from AIDS-related causes during the year.

Infectious diseases go hand in hand with poverty: overcrowding, lack of clean water and poor sanitation all encourage the spread of diseases, and lack of money reduces the access to drugs and treatment. The WHO estimates that nearly 2 million deaths worldwide each year are attributable to unsafe water, sanitation and hygiene.

In its report on infectious diseases published in 2000, the World Health Organisation highlighted the problem of antimicrobial resistance.

Although antimicrobial resistance is a natural phenomonon, the result of genetic mutation and Darwin's 'survival of the fittest', the effect has been amplified in recent years by the misuse of antimicrobials. Many treatments which were effective ten years ago are no longer so, and it is a sobering thought that there have been no new major developments in antimicrobial drugs for 30 years. Given that new drugs take at least ten years to develop and test, it is easy to see that a problem is looming. The WHO's director-general, Dr Gro Harlem Brundtland, quoted in the health pages of the CNN website (www.cnn.com/2000/HEALTH) said, 'We currently have effective medicines to cure almost every infectious disease, but we risk losing these valuable drugs and our opportunity to control infectious diseases.' Although it is commonly stated that the overuse of antimicrobials is the cause of the problem, it might be argued that it is actually the underuse that has done the damage since it is the pathogens that survive that cause the resistance.

Tourism also plays a part in the spread of diseases. The number of cases of malaria, yellow fever and other infectious diseases in developed countries is increasing as tourists catch the infections prior to returning to their own countries.

In 2000, the WHO carried out an analysis of the world's health by ranking countries by the life expectancy of their healthy population. This Disability Adjusted Life Expectancy (DALE) indicator placed Japan at the top (74.5 years) followed by Australia (73.2), France, Sweden, Spain, Italy and Greece. The bottom ten were all sub-Saharan African countries: Sierra Leone (25.9 years), Niger (29.1), Malawi (29.4), Zambia (30.3) and Botswana (32.3). AIDS killed 2.2 million Africans in 1999, compared to 300,000 deaths in 1989. In a separate ranking, based on the effectiveness of each country's health systems, France topped the table with the UK down in 18th place and the US in 37th. (Source: WHO reports 1999 and 2000.)

The World Health Organisation's website features data on health indicators for every country in the world. These highlight the differences in the standards of healthcare and the health problems in the rich and the poor countries of the world. You should take some time to look at the site in more detail. The data below will serve to give you a taster of the sort of issues that you should be aware of:

Country	Life expectancy	Per capita government expenditure at average exchange rate (US$) in 2000	Total health expenditure as a percentage of GDP, 2000	Dependency ratio
Japan	81.4 years	$2230	7.8%	48
UK	77.5 years	$1415	7.3%	53
India	61.0 years	$4	4.9%	62
Malawi	36.3 years	$5	7.6%	97

ROGUE DOCTORS

In recent years, the medical profession has been getting some bad press, particularly because of some well-publicised cases of 'rogue' doctors. You should make sure that you are aware of the problems at Alder Hey hospital, and at the Bristol Royal Infirmary. The name Harold Shipman, in particular, has been splashed across the front pages.

Dr Shipman

On Monday 31 January 2000, Dr Harold Shipman, a GP practising in Greater Manchester, was sentenced to life imprisonment for the murder of 15 of his patients. Police speculated that he could have been responsible for more than 300 other deaths. The question the medical profession has been asking itself is not 'why did he do it?' – there appears to be little motive apart from a desire to exert control – but 'how could it have gone unnoticed for such a long period of time?'

The case has been well documented and details can be found on the web sites of the national newspapers. The bigger issue is that of the monitoring and vetting of General Practitioners, particularly of those who run practices single-handedly. The problem only came to light when police were alerted by the daughter of one of his victims, who became suspicious after her mother's will had been clumsily altered by Shipman. What emerged was a catalogue of murders that had gone unnoticed for many years. All bar one of the victims had died in their own homes, a result of a diamorphine (the medical name for heroin) injection, administered under the pretext of taking a blood sample. The subsequent investigation revealed that Harold Shipman had a conviction for stockpiling pethidine, a drug, for his own use in 1975. He was able to obtain the diamorphine which he used to kill his patients in the same way, by analysing the medical records and making prescriptions for suitable patients which he then collected himself to store up for future use (Shipman had enough diamorphine to kill another 1000 patients).

Once he had decided on a victim, he amended the medical records so that there would be no suspicion surrounding the cause of death, and therefore no need for a post-mortem. One of the issues to arise from this is that of the so-called 'ash for cash' system whereby if the deceased is to be cremated, a second doctor's signature is required on the death certificate. However, although the second doctor is paid to do this, there is no requirement for this doctor to read the medical notes, perform an autopsy or to talk to relatives.

The General Medical Council (GMC), the body that registers and if necessary disciplines doctors, is now under pressure from the government to become more accountable and to improve its monitoring procedures. Amongst the measures being adopted or considered are:

- The establishment of a 'whistleblowing' hotline, through which suspicions could be relayed to the police or the GMC.
- The GMC to have a responsibility to inform health authorities of a GP's criminal and disciplinary past.
- A tightening of controls on the ability of a GP to hoard drugs – which would include preventing GPs collecting prescriptions for terminally ill patients, or collecting unused drugs from dead patients.
- A more thorough investigation of the cause of death by the second signatory on the death certificate.
- The establishment of computerised records of causes of death in order to identify any patterns that might be present.

Since the introduction of the GMC's emergency banning orders, brought in as a result of the Shipman case, about one doctor a week has been suspended.

HIV/AIDS

The World Health Organisation has estimated (World Health report 2002 – www.who.int/hiv/) that there are over 42 million people living with

HIV/AIDS. In that year, there were 5 million new infections, and over 3 million people died of HIV/AIDS or related infections. By far the biggest affected region is sub-Saharan Africa (29 million people with HIV/AIDS), where average life expectancy is now about 47 years, 15 years less than in the pre-HIV/AIDS era. The organisation estimates that 95 per cent of these infections are attributable to unsafe sex (compare this with a figure of 25 per cent in Eastern Europe). The global infection rate for adults is about 1 per cent (9 per cent for sub-Saharan Africa). The table below will give you an idea of how the rates of infection vary from country to country:

Country	Deaths in 1999	Total infected	Percentage of population affected
Botswana	24,000	290,000	36%
Lesotho	16,000	240,000	24%
South Africa	250,000	4.2 million	20%
Japan	150	10,000	0.02%
India	310,000	3.7 million	0.7%
UK	450	31,000	0.11%
USA	20,000	850,000	0.61%

Source: World Health Organisation

Most people who are infected with HIV are not aware of the fact and it is this that has caused the rapid growth of the problem. At the moment, there is no cure for HIV/AIDS, and no vaccine that is effective in protecting likely future sufferers. In February 2003, the US drugs company VaxGen announced the results of its large-scale trial of its AIDSVAX vaccine: the trial, involving 5400 volunteers, revealed that the vaccine appeared to have a protective effect among non-Caucasian populations, but this effect was small. At the moment, there are over twenty different vaccines being tested.

Measures that the WHO is advocating include:

- Mass-media health promotion campaigns
- School-based education targeted at males aged 10–18 years
- Treatment of mothers with HIV to prevent mother-to-child infections
- Dietary advice in order to delay progression of the virus.

POSTSCRIPT

If you have any comments or questions arising out of this book, the staff of MPW and I would be very happy to answer them. You can contact us at the addresses given below.

Good luck with your application to medical school!

James Burnett

MPW (Cambridge)
3/4 Brookside
Cambridge
CB2 1JE
Tel: 01223 350158
Fax: 01223 366429

MPW (London)
90/92 Queen's Gate
London
SW7 5AB
Tel: 020 7835 1355
Fax: 020 7225 2953

MPW (Birmingham)
38 Highfield Road
Edgbaston
Birmingham
B15 3ED
Tel: 0121 454 9637
Fax: 0121 454 6433

Table 1. Medical school admissions policies for 2004 entry

		Standard A-level offer	AS requirements	Subject preferences[1]	Retakes considered[2]	Type of course
LONDON MEDICAL SCHOOLS	Imperial College	ABB	A in the 4th AS	C and Biology or Chemistry A-level	C, and previously applied to IC Biology at A-level.	Integrated/Systems based
	King's	ABB	C grade	Either Biology or Chemistry A-level	B	Integrated/Systems based
	QMUL/Barts	ABB		C, 1st + 2nd science at A-level	C	Integrated/Systems based
	St George's	ABB	B grade	C, one at A-level	C	Integrated/Systems based
	Royal Free/UCL	ABB	No grade specified	B	B, BBC at first sitting	Integrated/Systems based
	Aberdeen	ABB	Not specified	A	No	Integrated/Systems based
	Belfast	AAA	AAB at A-level if extra AS grade A	B	A	Integrated/Systems based
OUTSIDE LONDON	Birmingham	AAB	Biology required at A/B	A	B	Integrated/Systems based
	Bristol	AAB	Not Specified	A	Grades AAB, at same time	Integrated/Systems based
	Dundee	ABB	AB at A-level, AB at AS-level	A	C	Integrated/Systems based
	Edinburgh	AAA/AAB	B if AAA at A-level, A if AAB at A-level	B, at least 1 other science at A-level	C	Integrated/Systems based
	Glasgow	AAB	No grade specified	A	C	Integrated/Systems based
	Leeds	AAB	Not specified	D	C	Integrated/Systems based
	Leicester/Warwick	AAB	No grade specified	B	C	Integrated/Systems based
	Liverpool	AAB	B grade (General Studies accepted)	C, two sciences A-level	C	Integrated/Systems based
	Manchester	AAB	No grade specified	D, + 1 or 2 other sciences at A-level	C	Integrated/Systems based
	Newcastle	AAB	Not specified	Either Chemistry or Biology	Yes	Integrated/Systems based

			Subject preferences		Retakes	
OUTSIDE LONDON	Nottingham	AAB	Not specified	E	C and previously held offer	Integrated/Systems based
	Sheffield	ABB	Recommend Chemistry, Biology, Maths or Physics, and one other subject	A, grades AB	Yes	Integrated/Systems based
	Southampton	AAB	Not specified	C, or A2 Chemistry	Yes, if 1 subject; if 2 subjects, see C	Integrated/Systems based
	St Andrews	ABB	Not specified	A – If Chem, Bio or Phys not at A2, GCSE necessary	Yes	Non-integrated/Subject based
	UWCM (Wales)	AAB		C, one of which to A-level	C, and previously applied to Wales. Biology at A-level	Integrated/Systems based
OXBRIDGE	Cambridge	AAA	Not specified	Chemistry at A or AS-level.	C	Non-integrated/Subject based
	Oxford	AAA	Not specified	A	C	Non-integrated/Subject based
NEW MEDICAL SCHOOLS	Brighton/Sussex Durham	ABB See Newcastle (AAB)	Bio, Chem to AS	C	Yes	Integrated/Systems based
	East Anglia	AAB, Access students encouraged to apply	Not specified	Biology	Yes	Integrated/Systems based
	Hull/York		B in AS Biology	B	Yes	Integrated/Systems based
	Keele	See Manchester				
	Peninsula	ABB–AAB	Not specified	C	No	Integrated/Systems based

1 Subject preferences key:
A Chemistry + one other science/mathematical subject, Biology preferred at A or AS-level; B A-level Chemistry + AS-level Biology; C Both Chemistry and Biology at least at AS-level; D Only Chemistry at A-level; E Chemistry and Biology at A-level.

2 Retakes key:
(Candidates will normally be expected to achieve AAA at second attempt); A Must have held an offer and have achieved BBB at first attempt. Will need AAA at second attempt; B Under exceptional circumstances, and if narrowly missed standard offer; C Extenuating circumstances.

Table 2. Medical school statistics – 2002 entry

	Applied	Interviewed	Offers	Accepted	Clearing	Graduates	Resits
LONDON MEDICAL SCHOOLS							
Imperial College	2488	1024	764	364	0	10	2
King's	2700*	1100	750	360	30	36	15
QMUL/Barts	1821	892	962	261	0	51	17
St George's	1350*	750	450	250	0	32	45
Royal Free/UCL	2362	1094	805	372	0	41	16
OUTSIDE LONDON							
Aberdeen	1115*	671	589	191	0	26	3
Belfast	551	37	324	183	0	9	3
Birmingham	1851	1300	1120	345	–	–	–
Bristol	2021	680	593	230	0	30	–
East Anglia	647	436	175	144	21	55	–
Dundee	1255	493	465	163	0	16	0
Edinburgh	1886*	40	513	215	0	6	0
Glasgow	1327	827	503	241	0	35	0
Leeds	1949	668	793	247	0	23	5
Leicester/Warwick	2513	1100	750	327	0	140	6
Liverpool	1516	1100	903	279	5	40	12
Manchester	1753*	974	789	352	0	51	12
Newcastle	2576	890	647	339	10	52	–
Peninsula	–	–	–	167	–	–	–
Nottingham	1806*	700	494	227	0	12	0
Sheffield	2243	992	700	249	0	45	11
Southampton	2356	213	540	200	14	37	–
St Andrews	492	45	336	109	10	3	7
UWCM (Wales)	1268*	820	643	329	6	16	3
OXBRIDGE							
Cambridge	1141*	1083	335	292	–	6	–
Oxford	788	705	174	158	0	3	0

* 2001 figures

83

Table 3. Interviews

	Length of typical interview	Number on panel	Composition of panel: drawn from[1]	Written element
LONDON MEDICAL SCHOOL				
Imperial College	15 mins	4	BCEFG	None
King's	15 mins	2	BCDF	20 min questionnaire before interview
OUTSIDE LONDON				
QMUL/Barts	15 mins	3	CEF	None
St George's	15 mins	3	BCDEFGJ	None
Royal Free/UCL	15—20 mins	3	ABCDEFGHJ	None
Aberdeen	20 mins	2/3	CFH	None
Belfast	15 mins	3	DFH	None
Birmingham	15 mins	3	BCDEFG	None
Bristol	15 mins	2	ABDCFG	None
Dundee	20 mins	2	FHJ	None
Edinburgh	30 mins	3	G	None
Glasgow	15 mins	2	ACDFG	None
Leeds	20 mins	3	ABCDE	None
Leicester/Warwick	15 mins	2	CE	None
Liverpool	15 mins	2	ACDFGI	None
Manchester	15 mins	4	CDFG	None
Newcastle	20 mins	2	ABCFGHIJ	None
Nottingham	15 mins	2	ABCDFGH	None
Sheffield	20 mins	3	CDEFIJ	None
Southampton	20 mins	2	ABCDFGH	None
St Andrews	20 mins	2/3	ABCDF	None
UWCM (Wales)	20 mins	2	ABCDEFGJ	None
OXBRIDGE				
Cambridge	At least 2 30-min interviews	2/3	BCF	2 hr MVAT test – see www.cam.ac.uk for details
Oxford	20—30 mins	2—4	CDF	1 1/4 hr test on English/data handling/analytical thinking
NEW MEDICAL SCHOOLS				
Durham	20 mins	2	ABCFGHIJ	None
East Anglia	30—45 mins	2	CD	None, but candidates given case history to discuss
Hull/York				
Keele	15 mins	4	CDFG	None

1. Key:
A Admissions Dean/Associate Dean; B Admissions Tutor; C Doctor from medical school; D Doctor from local area; E Medical student; F Academic staff; G Member of Admissions Committee; H Administrator; I Member of Trust Board; J Staff from other health professions.

APPENDIX A
MOCK INTERVIEW QUESTIONS

The importance of mock interviews – like mock exams – cannot be overemphasised. Most schools and independent sixth-form colleges are happy to arrange them, but, if this proves impossible, why not ask your parents or friends to help you? If you can get someone to record your answers on video, so much the better.

The questions set out below are designed to help your mock interviewer. Some of them have already been discussed; some will be new to you. At the end of the list there are five questions to help the interviewer check your posture, mannerisms, etc.

QUESTIONS FOR A MOCK INTERVIEW

Note to the interviewer: you should ask supplementary questions as appropriate.

1. Why do you want to be a doctor? (Supplementary: Are you sure you know what is involved?)

2. (If one of your parents is a doctor.) Presumably you chose medicine because of your father or mother?

3. What will you do if you don't get an offer from medical schools?

4. What evidence is there that you can cope with stress?

5. Why have you applied to this medical school?

6. What do you know about the course here?

7. Have you come along to an Open Day here?

8. What have you done to demonstrate your commitment to the community?

9. What makes a good doctor?

10. Why do you think you would make a good doctor?

11. What did the doctors you have spoken to think about medicine as a career?

12. What is the standard of health like in your area?

13. Why is the standard of health more varied in London/Scotland/ developing countries?

14. Are you interested in medical research?

15. What interests you about medicine? (Follow with questions about this area.)

16. What do you know about AIDS? Why is it so hard to treat?

17. What is the difference between a heart attack and a stroke?

18. What is the link between BSE and CJD?

19. What are the implications for doctors of an ageing population?

20. What problems do the elderly face?

21. What treatment can doctors offer to the very old?

22. What do you think of homeopathy/acupuncture?

23. How does diet affect health?

24. How does the environment affect health?

25. It was thought tuberculosis (TB) had been eradicated. Why do you think that the number of TB cases is now on the increase?

26. What roles can computers/technology play in medicine?

27. Tell me about a recent article on medicine/science that you have read. Explain it.

28. What are the main causes of ill health where you live?

29. What advances in medicine can we look forward to during the next ten/twenty/fifty years ?

30. What do you think have been the most significant developments in medicine during the last twenty/fifty/one hundred years?

31. What is the biggest threat to humanity over the next twenty/fifty years, from a medical viewpoint?

32. When was the NHS formed?

33. Have the reforms of the NHS been successful?

34. Should GPs/primary care groups act as fundholders?

35. What do you understand by the term rationing/postcode prescribing?

36. Do you think private practice by NHS consultants should be abolished?

37. Who is the Secretary of State for Health? What would you do if you had to take over this role?

38. Can anyone undertake cloning experiments in this country? What are the arguments for and against the cloning of humans?

39. Should the UK follow Holland's example and make euthanasia legal?

40. Is it right that the NHS should devote resources to sex change operations when there are long waiting lists for hip replacements?

41. Suppose that you were in charge of deciding which of two critically ill babies should have a life-saving operation. Imagine that there was not enough money to operate on both. How would you decide which baby to save?

42. Have you come across any examples of ethical problems associated with medicine?

43. What are your main interests? (The interviewer must follow up the answer with searching questions.)

44. How do you think you will be able to contribute to the life of the medical school?

45. What was the last book you read? Can you sum up the story in one minute?

46. What do you do in your spare time?

47. What is your favourite subject at A-level? What do you like about it?

48. What is your least favourite subject at A-level? What do you dislike about it?

49. (For retake candidates or those with disappointing GCSE results.) Why did you do badly in your A-levels/GCSEs?

50. What will you do if we decide not to offer you a place here?

51. Have you any questions for us?

QUESTIONS FOR THE INTERVIEWER TO ANSWER

1. Did the candidate answer in a positive, open and friendly way, maintaining eye contact for most of the time?

2. Was the candidate's posture such that you felt that he or she was alert, friendly and enthusiastic?

3. Was the candidate's voice pitched correctly; neither too loud nor too soft and without traces of arrogance or complacency?

4. Was the candidate free of irritating mannerisms?

5. Did the candidate's performance reassure you enough not to terrify you at the prospect that he or she could be your doctor in a few years?

APPENDIX B
THE INTERVIEW

THE PANEL

Most medical schools have so many candidates that they operate several interview panels in parallel. This means that your interview may not be chaired by the Dean but you will certainly have a senior member of the academic staff chairing the panel. He or she will normally be assisted by two or three others. Usually there are representatives of the clinical and pre-clinical staff and there may be a medical student on the board too. Sometimes a local GP is invited to join the panel. Details of the format of the interview panels can be found in Table 3 (page 84).

While you can expect the interviewers to be friendly, it is possible that one of them may use an aggressive approach. Don't be put off by this; it is a classic interview technique and will usually be balanced by a supportive member of the panel.

QUESTIONNAIRES

A number of medical schools have introduced a written component to the interview. Some, such as Nottingham and Southampton, ask for a form or an essay to be sent to them prior to the interview. Others, such as St George's and GKT, give each candidate a written exercise on the day of the interview. Bear in mind that a candidate who performs well in the interview, displays the necessary academic and personal qualities, and is genuinely suited to medicine, is unlikely to be rejected on the basis of the written element.

DRESS, POSTURE AND MANNERISMS

You should dress smartly for your interview, but you should also feel comfortable. You will not be able to relax if you feel over-formal. For men, a jacket with a clean shirt and tie is ideal. Women should avoid items of clothing or jewellery which jar: no big earrings, plunging neck lines or short skirts. Men should not wear earrings, white socks or loud ties, or have (visible) piercings. They should avoid unconventional hairstyles: no mohicans or skinheads.

Your aim must be to give an impression of good personal organisation and cleanliness. Make a particular point of your hair and fingernails – you never see a doctor with dirty fingernails. Always polish your shoes before an interview, as this type of detail will be noticed. Don't go in smelling strongly of garlic, aftershave or perfume.

You will be invited to sit down, but don't fall back expansively into an armchair, cross your legs and press your fingertips together in an impersonation of Sherlock Holmes. Sit slightly forward in a way that allows you to be both comfortable and alert.

Make sure that you arrive early and well prepared for the interview.

Try to achieve eye contact with each member of the panel and as much as possible address your answer directly to the panel member who asked the question (glancing regularly at the others), not up in the air or to a piece of furniture. Most importantly, try to relax and enjoy the interview. This will help you to project an open, cheerful personality.

Finally, watch out for irritating mannerisms. These are easily checked if you videotape a mock interview. The interviewers will not listen to what you are saying if they are all watching to see when you are next going to scratch your left ear with your right thumb.

APPENDIX C
ADVICE ON REVISION

ACTIVE REVISION

Revision technique makes sense when you understand that revision is really the same as rehearsal. You rehearse a school play so that all goes well on the night. Reading through the script and watching other productions on video may help but the crucial activity is rehearsal itself. First you rehearse short scenes with the script in your hand, then whole acts and finally the complete play on stage in costume. So it is with exam preparation: everything must lead up to the performance. Everything you do must contribute to your ability to answer the exam questions effectively, in the exam hall, on the appointed day and in the time allowed.

All revision should be active. The student who spends hours reading and re-reading notes, perhaps with the highlighter pen in hand, is demonstrating the art of passive revision (which, in turn, leads to angst in August). Active revision means testing yourself on all parts of the syllabus.

1. Read a section of your notes.
2. Write out a page of revision notes, including key definitions, facts and diagrams.
3. Learn the revision notes.
4. An hour later, try to write out another set of revision notes, from memory. Compare them with the original, and correct them.
5. A day later, write out the notes, again from memory.
6. Repeat as often as necessary.
7. Use past paper questions, under timed conditions, every day. Either get them marked by a teacher, or use your revision notes to correct them.

The stairway to exam heaven

Step 1 – Planning the programme
Revision needs to be planned and the plan needs to be based on the syllabus for each subject you are taking. Make a list of the topics and allocate time to each one in a programme that allows for a period of revision each day between now and the last exam. Allow spare time for contingencies and for relaxation.

Run the finished plan past your teachers and finally publish it by sticking a copy in some prominent place where your parents can see it. This serves two purposes: it helps to convince them that you are serious about revision and the programmed breaks give you official time off. One word of warning: don't spend too long planning your programme.

Step 2 – Understand and learn
Before you can rehearse a play you need a copy of the script, an understanding of the character you are playing and you must have learned the words and stage directions. The same principles apply to revision. The first step in revising any topic is to check the relevant pages of the syllabus, read your notes, look through your homework and model answers and check that you really understand the material. Then identify and learn the sections that need to be remembered (including formulae that may be given in formulae sheets). This is where those famous summary cards can come in useful. The act of summarising your notes on file cards can help you remember facts. You can also ask a friend or parent to test you using the cards. Other learning techniques (such as mind maps) may be useful to you.

Step 3 – Exam practice
This is the key, crucial, vital revision activity and the only proof that your revision has been worthwhile. Attempt real exam questions from the syllabus you are studying (watch for syllabus changes) under self-imposed exam conditions (no books, no music and with the clock running). To be fair, you will find this difficult at the start and you may need help from your notes and more time than the examiner allows, but keep pushing towards the ideal.

Step 4 – Self-check
After each practice session you need to mark your work. Be tough on yourself: is your answer accurate, neat and easy to read? Have you

answered the question? For example, did you define something you were asked to describe? (Examiners have their own special vocabulary, and they like you to pay attention to it.) Above all, are your answers complete and correct? This may be easy to check if, for example, you have practised a multiple-choice paper for which you have answers.

For other questions you may need access to the examiners' mark scheme (which your school or college will have) or a model answer. Even then, you may not be able to find an answer or, having found it, you may not understand why it is correct. If so, you will need the help of your teacher. Don't be shy; most teachers are only too happy to help a student who is revising conscientiously. Don't forget that your good grades will reflect well on your teacher and on your school.

Step 5 – More of the same
You need to repeat steps 3 and 4 for all topics in all subjects and with all question types. The number of questions you attempt at each session needs to increase until you can concentrate for the full duration of the real exam – perhaps as long as three hours. With luck, the areas of difficulty identified in the self-check will get fewer and your confidence will grow. If this isn't happening, you may need some extra help from your teacher or, if that is impossible, from a tutor outside school.

A few last words of advice
Effective revision is tough and will certainly involve sacrifices, but hard work now is well worthwhile if it prevents low grades, lost places and the possibility of having to abandon cherished career plans. Most exams can be retaken but you'll have to revise effectively for the retake, so why not do it now?

APPENDIX D
SUGGESTIONS FOR FURTHER
RESEARCH

COURSES

Insight Into Medicine
Small group, two-day courses for sixth-formers in a hospital which allows students to work with doctors, technicians, nurses and volunteer patients to explore the theory, diagnosis and treatment of specific medical conditions such as heart disease. Contact MPW on 0121 454 9637.

Medisix
Intensive residential course at Nottingham University School of Medicine, consisting of a series of lectures covering a wide range of medical subjects. There is also a casualty simulation exercise.

Telephone 01509 235879 for details.

PUBLICATIONS

Careers in Medicine

Learning Medicine, Professor Peter Richards (formerly Dean and Professor of Medicine at St Mary's Hospital Medical School), BMJ Publishing Group, Tavistock Square, London WC1H 9JR.

Careers in Medicine, Dentistry and Mental Health, Judith Humphries, Kogan Page, 120 Pentonville Road, London N1 9JN.

A Career in Medicine, ed. Harvey White, Royal Society of Medicine Press (www.roysocmed.ac.uk).

The Insider's Guide to Medical Schools, Urmston and Calvert, BMJ Publications.

Medical Science – General

The Oxford Illustrated Companion to Medicine, ed. Stephen Lock, John M Last and George Dunea, OUP.

Oxford Companion to the Body, Blakemore & Jennett, OUP

The White Death – A History of Tuberculosis, Thomas Dormandy, Hambledon.

The Trouble with Medicine, Dr Melvin Konner, BBC Worldwide Ltd.

How We Die, Sherwin Nuland, Vintage.

How We Live, Sherwin Nuland, Vintage.

Why We Age, Steven N Austab, John Wiley.

The Human Brain: A Guided Tour, Susan Greenfield, Weidenfeld & Nicolson.

Plague, Pox and Pestilence: Disease in History, Kenneth Kiple, Weidenfeld & Nicolson.

Medicine and Culture, Lynn Payer, Victor Gollancz.

The Secret Family, David Bodanis, Simon & Schuster.

Pain – the Science of Suffering, Patrick Wall, Weidenfeld & Nicolson.

Medicine – a History of Healing, ed. Roy Porter, Michael O'Mara Books.

The Greatest Benefit to Mankind, Roy Porter, Fontana.

Practical Medical Ethics, Seedhouse and Lovett, John Wiley.

Body Story, Dr David Willham, Channel 4 Books.

Catching Cold, Pete Davies, Michael Joseph/Penguin.

Flu, Gina Kolata, Pan.

Human Instinct, Robert Winston, Bantam.

Genetics

The Sequence, Kevin Davies, Weidenfeld & Nicolson.

Clone, Gina Kolata, Allen Lane/Penguin Press.

Who's Afraid of Human Cloning?, Gregory and Pence, Rowman and Littlefield.

Genome, Matt Ridley, Fourth Estate.

The Blind Watchmaker, Richard Dawkins, Penguin.

The Language of the Genes, Steve Jones, Flamingo.

Y: The Descent of Man, Steve Jones, Bantam.

Medical Ethics

Causing Death and Saving Lives, Jonathan Glover, Penguin.

Medical Practice

Medic One On Scene, Dr Heather Clark, Virgin.

Patients' Choice, David Cook, Hodder & Stoughton.

A Damn Bad Business: The NHS Deformed, Jeremy Lee, Victor Gollancz.

Patient: The True Story of a Rare Illness, Ben Watt, Viking.

Higher Education Entry

University and College Entrance: The Official Guide, UCAS.

Degree Course Offers, Brian Heap, Trotman & Co.

How To Complete Your UCAS Form, Tony Higgins, MPW Guides/ Trotman & Co.

Getting into Oxford and Cambridge, MPW Guides/Trotman & Co.

The Mature Students' Guide, Trotman & Co.

WEB SITES

All of the medical schools have their own web sites, and there are numerous useful and interesting medical sites. These can be found using search engines. Particularly informative sites include:

World Health Organisation: www.who.int

Department of Health: www.open.gov.uk/doh

British Medical Association: www.bma.org.uk

Student BMJ: www.studentbmj.com

UCAS: www.ucas.com

EXAMINERS' REPORTS

The examining boards provide detailed reports on recent exam papers, including mark schemes and specimen answers. Schools are sent these every year by the boards. They are useful when analysing your performance in tests and mock examinations. If your school does not have copies, they can be obtained from the boards themselves. The examining boards' addresses are available from schools or libraries.

APPENDIX E
USEFUL ADDRESSES

STUDYING IN THE UK

Carol Baverstock
Head of Admissions
Kings College
Aberdeen University
Aberdeen
AB24 3FX

Mr S Wisener
Admissions Officer
Queen's University Belfast
Northern Ireland
BT7 1NN

Professor Chris Lote
Admissions Tutor
The Medical School
Birmingham
B15 2TT

Professor Jon Cohen
Brighton and Sussex Medical School
Mithras House
Lewes Road
Brighton
BN2 4AT

Miss Pat Bye
Admissions Officer
Faculty of Medicine
University of Bristol

Senate House
Tyndall Avenue
Bristol
BS8 1TH

Head of Cambridge Admissions Office
Kellet Lodge
Tennis Court Road
Cambridge
CB2 1QJ

Mrs Pam Clark
Assistant Registrar
(Recruitment and Admissions)
University of Wales College of Medicine
Heath Park
Cardiff
CF14 4XN

Mr Gordon Black
Admissions Officer
Admissions and Student Recruitment
University of Dundee
Dundee
DD1 4HN

Professor Sam Leinster
Dean
School of Medicine
University of East Anglia
Norwich
NR4 7TJ

Dr D M Thompson
Associate Dean for Admissions
The Medical School
Teviot Place
Edinburgh
EH8 9DF

Anne Cooney
Admissions Secretary
Medical School
University of Glasgow
Glasgow
G12 8QQ

Connie Cullen
Hull York Medical School
York University
Heslington
York
YO10 5DD

Dr David Dawson
Sub-Dean for Admissions
University of Leeds Medical School
Worsley Building
Leeds
LS2 9JT

Dr Kevin West
Senior Tutor for Admissions
Maurice Shock Medical Science Building
University Road
Leicester
LE1 9HN

Jane Goldberg
Admissions Officer
Faculty of Medicine
Duncan Building
Daulby
Liverpool
L69 3GA

London

Martyn Annis
Assistant Registrar (Admissions)
Student Admissions Office
King's College London
Hodgkin Building
Guy's Campus
London
SE1 1UL

David Gibbon
Admissions Officer
School of Medicine
Imperial College of Science, Technology & Medicine
London
SW7 2AZ

Dr Brenda Cross
Sub-Dean and Faculty Tutor
Royal Free & University College Medical School
University College London
Faculty of Life Sciences
Gower Street
London
WC1E 6BT

Ms Hannah Eno
Bart's & The London School of Medicine & Dentistry
Turner Street
London
E1 2AD

Ms Caroline Persaud
Admissions Officer
St George's Hospital School of Medicine
Cranmer Terrace
London
SW17 0RE

Mrs Linda Harding
Admissions Officer
University of Manchester Medical School
Stopford Building
Oxford Road
Manchester
M13 9PT

Mrs Pat Carslisle
Admissions Officer
The Medical School
Framlington Place
Newcastle upon Tyne
NE2 4HH

Ms Kate Squires
Admissions Officer
University of Nottingham Medical School
Queen's Medical Centre
Nottingham
NG7 2UH

Dr Catherine Hawkins
Pre-Clinical Studies Office
Medical Sciences Teaching Centre
South Parks Road
Oxford
OX1 3RE

Miss L Snowdon
Peninsula Medical School
ITTC Tamar Science Park
Davy Road
Plymouth
PL6 8BX

Miss A Skrypczak
Medical Admissions Officer
Faculty of Medicine
Beech Hill Road
Sheffield
S10 2RX

Dr Jenny Skidmore
Admissions Tutor
School of Medicine
Biomedical Sciences Building
Bassett Crescent East
Southampton
SO16 7PX

Dr David Jackson
Medical Admissions Officer
Admissions Application Centre
79 North Street
St Andrews
Fife
KY16 9AJ

ACCESS TO MEDICINE COURSE

Derek Holmes
The College of West Anglia
Tennyson Avenue
King's Lynn
Norfolk
PE30 2QW
01553 761 144 (Ext 309)

STUDYING OUTSIDE THE UK

Royal College of Surgeons in Ireland
123 St Stephen's Green
Dublin 2
Eire
www.rcsi.ie

Margaret Lambert
St George's University School of Medicine
C/o One East Main Street
Bay Shore
New York
Sgu_info.sgu.edu
0800 169 9061 (from UK)

M & D Europe (UK) Ltd
Medicine & Dentistry Degree Admission Services
Suite 579
28 Old Brompton Road
London
SW7 3SS
0871 717 1291
www.readmedicine.com
(For English-language medicine courses in the Czech Republic)